AID FROM ABOVE
(Auxilium Desuper)

Inside My Veiled World as a Flight Nurse

Kurtis Bell, RN, CFRN

Isabell Fromme Publishing

Aid From Above (Axilium Desuper): Inside My Veiled World as a Flight Nurse
Copyright © 2019 by Kurtis Bell

Cover Design by Linda Kosarin/The Art Department
Typeset by Raymond Luczak

All rights reserved, including the right of reproduction in whole or in part in any form.

For more information, please contact:
Web: www.kurtisbell.com
Email: anotherson@kurtisbell.com

Published by Isabell Fromme Publishing

Paperback: 978-0-9995823-4-3
Hardcover: 978-0-9995823-5-0
Ebook: 978-0-9995823-6-7
Kindle: 978-0-9995823-7-4

Distributed by Ingram Content Group
Printed in the United States

First Edition 2019

Table of Contents

Acknowledgement i
Author's Note iii
Preface: Let Me Tell You 1
Chapter 1: Another Day 3
Chapter 2: Don't Lose Your Head 19
Chapter 3: Auxilium Desuper 33
Chapter 4: Aeromedical 41
Chapter 5: Nursing 49
Chapter 6: The Burn 54
Chapter 7: Go to the Light 65
Chapter 8: The Phoenix Open 73
Chapter 9: The News 83
Chapter 10: Personalities - Abbreviated 93
Chapter 11: Airfield Crash 100
Chapter 12: Shit Happens 108
Chapter 13: PR 128
Chapter 14: Don't Lose Face 133
Chapter 15: Drowned in the Moment 146
Chapter 16: The Antler Guy 155
Chapter 17: Out of Limits 165

Chapter 18: Laura	185
Chapter 19: The Life, Love, and Rumors	189
Chapter 20: The Answer is NO	193
Chapter 21: Don't Tell Anyone	196
Chapter 22: Oh, Crikey	204
Chapter 23: Rick Heape	216
Chapter 24: Change	222
Chapter 25: Poor Ol' Cow	225
Chapter 26: Didn't Read the Book	231
Chapter 27: Matt Uhl	245
Chapter 28: Get Pumping	250
Chapter 29: EMS	257
Chapter 30: The World of Transport	262
Chapter 31: Going Down	274
Chapter 32: The Heartbreak	281
Chapter 33: Outcomes and Results	300
Memoriae	309
Author's Bio	310

Acknowledgement

I wish to dedicate this book to the countless multitude of people that have dedicated their lives to the care of other human beings from tragedy to wellness all over the world. It is through their commitment that many survive. More specifically, to those responders whose unsaid motto is, "Risking ours to save yours." They do it completely without thought of self or pursuit of glory, they do it because it is in their makeup. It is what makes them who they are.

I also wish to make a special thank you to a long-time colleague of mine who sparked me to write this. He is a great friend that I consider a brother.

James Locke, RN, MSN, CFRN

Author's Note

All of the scenarios presented in this book are actual events from my career with Native American Air Ambulance from 1997 to 2010. The names of all of the patients or victims have been changed due to strict HIPPA laws. The names of my colleagues are real.

The profession of medical flight transport is one steeped in wonder. When it is shown in medical documentaries and literature, it is often seen in a blinding light of glory and high magnitude. In reality, it is a somewhat veiled, very personal world that is often kept hidden for a reason. Though it is open for any to observe and the participants are not shy or elusive about what they do, it is kept discreet for the protection of the doctor's, nurse's, and medic's own humanity. Just as a curtain is drawn around a patient in a trauma room, there are some things that are private and not meant for those not directly involved. That includes the emotions and feelings of the medical professionals trained in this arena. Above all they are very human. Many of the things they do and endure are not easily understandable to those that are not familiar with that world.

It's hard to explain the anguish of telling a parent you

could not save their child or listen to the wails of people as you work on their loved one. Without being immersed in that experience, it's difficult to appreciate that reality.

We are not angels from above, we are merely humans from above.

With this book, I try to draw back that veil for just a moment so you can see the impact that world had on me after two decades in flight. I would like to stress that this is only from my point of view and not intended to represent any of the thousands of other aeromedical personnel formerly or currently working in this field. Some of the finest human beings I've ever had the privilege to know and associate with. Once family, always family!

Preface
LET ME TELL YOU

With the inevitable passage of time, "dreams of what could be" become "memories of what was."

I'm now in my sixties. This evening I grab the handle of my ambulance door and step inside, preparing for my shift. Currently, my full-time job is as an RN working on a ground Critical Care Nurse Transport unit with a company in Phoenix, Arizona. I also keep a part-time position with a medical flight company on the side. Flight nursing is in my blood, but these days my body is better suited to staying on the ground most of the time.

My EMT partner, Mateo Romero, climbs in the driver's seat beside me. It's early in his healthcare career. In a few months, he'll be going to school for his paramedic certification. He has the unenviable task of joining me throughout a twelve-hour shift, three days a week. He's a curious sort and because of that is quite intelligent. He knows that I have over twenty years in emergency flight transport. I don't recall him ever specifically asking about my past flight experiences, and to his credit, he never complains and listens attentively when I talk about it.

Mateo has an interest of possibly pursuing a career in

flight after obtaining his paramedic certificate. As many new medics and nurses do. So, hearing the stories I tell keeps him entertained, especially on those long shifts when we don't get many, if any, calls. The critical care transport business is one of wait: wait for the call, wait, it's coming, wait, okay you got a call. Then after you finish with that one, wait some more, wait for it, wait. But when you do get the call, you often get tested. Not only of your abilities but often your patience.

Mr. Romero is one of the best partners I've ever had and a patient listener. Here are some of the things I told him.

Chapter 1
ANOTHER DAY

I was walking out to the helicopter at three o'clock one morning. It was not cold out. It was not even cool, not even a little. It was August in Phoenix, Arizona. It's not cool out anytime in August in Phoenix. In fact, it's still 95 degrees Fahrenheit. As soon as I came out of the hangar door, I lit up a cigarette. It was about two hundred feet to the helicopter. I could get a couple of puffs in before I left. It was not that I really had to have it, but it had become an unconscious routine. A habit that I didn't really think about. I only got a couple of drags on it before I was fifty-feet from the aircraft, too close by protocol to smoke, but it was enough.

Walking across the tarmac out to the helicopter, it was quiet. Only because it was three in the morning. It was dark except for a few lights illuminating the taxiways. At that time, I worked for Native American Air Ambulance and our helicopter's pad was back by the fence, where there was a lamp highlighting her like a stage light. She was sitting a safe distance behind another medical helicopter, that of our competitor. That helicopter was yellow with black stripes. Normally this area was quite busy with student pilots from the school based here and private pilots checking out their aircraft, running them up and taxiing out. But not now. It was dark, deserted, and so quiet you could hear coyotes in the distance wailing up a storm. It gave you the feeling that you were the last humans on earth.

When we approached the helipad, Bud, our pilot, had already done his required "walk around" inspection and was getting in to fire up the helicopter. Brian, my paramedic teammate, was beside me, walking out carrying the drug box. I had my clipboard and a water bottle. Coming up to the nose of the aircraft, we split up. He goes to the left door and I go around to climb in the right door that's behind the pilot. In a helicopter, the pilot-in-command sits on the right side.

As a registered nurse, I am one of the three-part team that staffs a medical helicopter in Native American Air Ambulance. Obviously, all have a pilot as one of the team but other companies and other states staff their medical helicopters differently. Some staff with a doctor on board, others may have a respiratory therapist accompany the nurse, some may have two paramedics and some may have a specialty team, like neonatal. Our company's medical team always had at least one RN accompanied, primarily, with a paramedic or possibly another RN.

Our helicopter was a Bell 206 L-3 Long Ranger that we have affectionately named "Little Girl." She was the first helicopter that Native American Air Ambulance, or NAAA, obtained when we first started helicopter missions. Before that, NAAA started out just providing fixed-wing transports with two Jet Stream twin-engine aircrafts. The "wings" on a helicopter are the large blades on top. They rotate to provide lift, hence they are known as "rotor-wing" aircraft. On the other hand, on an airplane, the wings are fixed in place, hence their name, "fixed-wing." Later when the company grew and added another helicopter, it was also a Bell 206, but it sat on high skids. Little Girl sat on low skids that made her look smaller and more petite. Personally, I thought she looked more sporty and sexy than the other helicopter. The low skids were how she got her name "Little Girl." Her real name was N206AZ. That was printed on her side and how she was known to the Federal Aviation Administration. But to us, she was just Little Girl. It is widely accepted that air and sea vessels are always referred to in the feminine. I don't really know why, but I have my suspicions. Historically, the first to command these vessels were men.

As soon as Brian and I got in, we secured our equipment then buckled up. I put my headset on and adjusted the mic to my bottom lip. We did a quick look around to make sure all was good and then clicked the button on our headset cord to let Bud know we were good to go.

With that Bud said, "Coming hot," and the engine started to wind up. The blades, ever so slowly, started to rotate around faster and faster, and you heard a *click, click, click, click, click* of the fuel igniters until, suddenly, a whoosh of the Jet A fuel firing. It took a moment until the blades were spinning at the required speed, with the pilot adjusting the throttle to obtain the right RPMs. Bud allowed her to run for a minute to stabilize while he finished his mandatory pre-flight checks. While he did that, I wrote down basic information and got my chart started. Brian took this time to finish strapping up his boots and zipping up his flightsuit.

Our dispatch was for a motor vehicle accident, known as an MVA, north of our position on Interstate 17. Before Bud actually pulled up on the "Collective," the level on his left that, as Bud put it, "made the trees get smaller," he checked in with, "All secure?" We clicked back affirmatively and Little Girl started to rise into the air like a carnival ride. We were off!

Bud is an older gentleman, mid-sixties, getting close to retirement with a long career as a helicopter pilot, reaching back into the Vietnam War era. Sparse grey hair covered with a hat sitting off kilter and a belly that protrudes through his partially zipped flightsuit portrays a manner of "Been there, done that, and now I'm just going to do it again." Like a good grandpa, I don't think I have ever heard a bitter word come from him. The most laid back, nonchalant, devil-may-care pilot that I have ever known. By this time, I have flown with well over fifty pilots. His attitude to life may have been casual but his attention to safety was well focused and deliberate. In fact, Bud had a tendency to fly a good bit higher than most for safety. As he put it, "The higher you go, the less likely you are to hit a granite cloud." His way of saying a mountain. The standing joke was that Bud flew so high that he was on a first name basis with NASA's Shuttle pilots and probably knew them all personally. Well, he just might have. Bud was one of those people that everybody knew. For one thing, he'd been around for a considerable time in this industry, but also because of his outgoing personality and lifestyle. Forth of July party ... Bud's house. New Year's Eve party ... Bud's house. His wife was a registered nurse and was as sociable as he was. Their social network was pretty extensive, even before modern technology.

I, on the other hand, am much less sociable. Not intentionally, just by my personality and circumstance. I'm married with two boys and a dog. When I'm not at work, I'm at home trying to catch up with family life. I try to keep my lives separate. I don't want to be distracted at work worrying about what's going on at home. I don't want to carry home what happens at work. My wife, and especially my kids, end up with a sanitized version of what I see at work. *No, I don't want you climbing up on that wall. Don't you know what I just saw because of something like that? No, don't do that. The last kid I flew on did something like that. Stay away from there.* It took me awhile to realize I wasn't letting my own family fully enjoy life because of all the freak accidents I would see at different scenes and the consequences of them at hospitals. Eventually, I relaxed, but work still always remained in the back of my mind when I was home.

I heard Bud key up the radio, "Dispatch, Native 5, lifting to the scene, ETA twelve minutes." Our particular base designation for the company was Native 5. This was the fifth rotor-wing base the company put up since it started doing helicopter missions in 1997. Because of the name, Native American Air Ambulance, many people thought that we only responded to or transported Native Americans or we only employed Native Americans. But Native American Air Ambulance was a privately-owned air ambulance service that did everything all the other air ambulance services did; no different. We employed anyone who was qualified. Rick, the owner, named it that because he was part Native American, though you wouldn't know it to look at him.

"Copy, Native 5, lifting. Location Interstate 17, mile marker two-forty-three. Single vehicle rollover. Ground contact Engine thirty-two," dispatch replied.

"Single vehicle rollover, huh?" Brian said with a look that said, "What's this going to be?"

I glanced up at him and shrugged. A single vehicle rollover

can be as serious as someone thrown several feet out of the car with massive injuries or as simple as someone who's been in an accident but is up walking around without any complaints. Both are possible, as well as anything in between.

A rollover MVA is just one of several classifications that automatically initiates a trauma response. It's in the classification known as "trauma by mechanism." There are a few in this class. If a vehicle rolls over, or if the victim sustains a loss of consciousness, known as a positive LOC, if someone is ejected from the vehicle, or if someone else in the vehicle is killed, then it is automatically considered a trauma. The reason behind that is, because of the dynamics involved with the mechanism of the event, there is a possibility for someone to be seriously injured and maybe not know it. Even if you are able to get up and walk around without any complaints or obvious injuries, you may still have an internal injury that you're not aware of and should be treated like a real trauma until a qualified physician examines you. You could have bleeding in the brain or a fractured spine and not even know it. There are other mechanisms in this class, like falling from a height greater than ten feet onto a hard surface, with or without obvious injury and so on. Which all boils down to, you never know what you're going to walk into when you get one of these calls.

I glanced out of the window to get my bearings as to where we were right then. I noticed the dark, middle-of-the-night peacefulness of the ground going by, just slightly lit by the half moon in the clear sky. Everything had a light blue tint to it, everything that I could see anyway. It gave the impression that it was cool out there on the ground. But I knew better.

It wasn't long when I started seeing the lights of Black

Canyon City below. A small town just north of Phoenix. As I looked up I could see a cluster of red and blue police lights flickering on the highway and knew that was our scene. We were still a few minutes away so I started to prepare to land. I pulled out about six inches of three-inch-wide cloth tape and placed it on my right thigh. I use this to write down information I would get on the scene from the ground crews. Then I donned a pair of elastic gloves.

Bud keyed up the radio again. This time it was set to the channel the ground crew was using. He gave them our ETA and requested landing instructions. The ground crew would give him instructions as to where they wanted him to land, provide wind conditions, and note any obstacles or hazards in the area. Sometimes they would add some patient information in order to give the medical crew a heads up. This was not one of those times.

They wanted us to land on the highway just south of the ambulance that was south of the accident site. The highway was already pretty well blocked by dirt and gravel debris from the roadsides and vehicle parts as well as the vehicle itself, but just to be sure, there were two police cruisers north of the accident, lights flashing, blocking oncoming traffic from this side of the divided highway.

Bud did an obligatory circle around the scene to get a good look at the landing site and any obstacles that he could see that were not mentioned. What you can see from the air is of course entirely different than what you can see on the ground. Plus he was gauging wind speed and direction and planning his approach to the landing spot. There are many things to take into account when choosing an approach and speed of descent to a landing zone. All of which were just instinctive for Bud.

At that point, Brian and I were looking out our respective sides of the helicopter, prepared to alert Bud if we saw anything that would prevent a safe landing. This was at the top of our list. Landing a helicopter in a place that was not designed for that purpose always involves risks. The wind the helicopter was generating may blow objects into the site or may blow them away dangerously close to other things and people. Wires may be in the path of decent that were not noticed by the ground crew farther away. The landing surface could be oddly angled and off-kilter, making setting down perilous or impossible. Not to mention you were seriously close to the ground and so if the engine even hiccupped, things could get really ugly really fast. That was one of the things that made this job a little precarious, but also fun. Along with the different medical situations we'd walk into, the unusual flying situations we would find ourselves in kept our work adventurous and exciting. However, any sane person would question that idea of fun.

Once our skids touched the ground, I looked at my watch and marked down the time on the tape on my leg. Bud gave us the "all-clear" once Little Girl had settled. Brian and I grabbed what we were going to take with us. With the declaration, "We're out," we opened the doors. Most of our emergency calls we stayed "hot," which meant that Bud would not shut down the helicopter. It stayed running, ready to go.

As I walked into the controlled chaos, I looked for where the patient was and took in all that I could about the scene. Like 99% of the scenes we arrive at, this one already had firefighters and paramedics attending to the patient. They could be at the vehicle, still trying to extricate the victim from the car or they could be by the vehicle, treating the patient or they could already be in the back of the ambulance awaiting our arrival.

Generally, by this time they already had the patient secured on a long backboard and had an IV inserted. In this case, I was directed by one of the firefighters to the ambulance, where they had the patient.

Because this was a potential trauma patient and this scene was quite a distance from the nearest Level One trauma center, the ground crew determined it to be prudent to use a helicopter for rapid transport.

There is no set rule in our company as to who does what when it came to the nurse and medic. When we work, we just consider each other teammates who strive for a single goal: getting the job done. Most of the time, unless we're both busy treating the patient, I would get a report from the ground medic about what happened and what's been done for the patient. Along with what personal information they know about the patient like name, date of birth, medical history, and allergies. In the meantime, my medic would be doing his assessment of the patient and getting them attached to our monitors and ready to go.

We came out of the ambulance with the gurney, accompanied by two medics and a firefighter, and headed to Little Girl sitting there patiently waiting for us. Everyone has been trained on the proper procedure for approaching a hot helicopter and how to load one. But I knew Brian was watching everything very closely to make sure no one forgot anything, as was I. If anything went wrong, we were responsible. I hurried ahead of them so I could get the door opened and the inside ready. I turned around to see that everybody was safe. Four of us lifted the backboard from the gurney and slid the patient inside while one person held the gurney from rolling back to the tail of the aircraft. It's a standing rule that if you let go of the gurney, it will always roll back to the tail, the danger zone. No reason why. Hell, the slope of the road may even be going in the opposite direction. But for some unearthly reason, once the gurney is let free, the damn thing always goes for the tail-rotor. Unbelievable.

When loading a patient, a flight crew member always stands as far back as anyone is allowed to go toward the tail of the aircraft. The tail rotor spins so fast it can be hard to see. That's why there is a red arrow on tail booms pointing to the rear of the aircraft with the word "danger" in it. If anyone forgets and tries to go that way past them, they are abruptly stopped and turned around. Once the patient was strapped and locked in, we thanked the crews for helping. Watched to make sure they left the site toward the front so Bud could see and count everyone that came up. Once everyone was away, Brian went around to get secured in the helicopter and started putting equipment where we wanted it. I waited for him to get in then shut and secured the door before going around myself. There is usually a firefighter or police officer standing well behind the landing zone to guard the tail-rotor area from anyone inadvertently walking up. My usual practice is to give him a thumb up and a wave of appreciation before climbing in. It's respectful. That routine of mine is important to remember.

As soon as I buckled in and plugged in my headset, I let Bud know that we were good to go. At that point we both took our attention away from the patient briefly to concentrate on the ascent. When it came to the riskiest times of flight, this was the second on the list for most of the same reasons as landing. Up we came and then off we went.

This was a common type of patient we attended to from a rollover MVA. It was the middle of the night and this single person in the car became drowsy and wandered off the edge of the road. He snapped awake and over corrected the vehicle, making it flip over as the tires dug into the soft shoulder. He was thirty-six years old and restrained with seatbelts. He had a positive LOC, or loss of consciousness, but regained consciousness before EMS arrived. He wasn't complaining much, but said his back was hurting. There were no obvious injuries found on him except for the slightly red mark across his hips from the seatbelt, but he was considered a trauma because he complained of back pain which could indicate a spinal injury and enough mechanism was involved that he needed to be taken to a trauma unit for evaluation. With the report I received and after evaluating the patient for ourselves and feeling reasonably comfortable that he was stable, Brian could just monitor his vital signs and gaze out the window. I concentrated on the ever-important paperwork and started writing his chart. There was not much conversing with the patient because he couldn't hear us very well nor us him. The flight crew had on headsets so we could talk to each other via the intercom, but the patient just had in ear plugs because of the noise.

We landed on the helipad of John C. Lincoln Hospital, the closest trauma facility, about sixteen minutes from the scene by helicopter. While the blades were slowing down, I got out and opened the patient side door. As soon as we were ready, I motioned for the security guard with the gurney to come up. Minutes later we were in the trauma room with the team all converging on the patient all at once. Over the clamor and seeming chaos, I gave report that explained the patient and situation to the doctor and trauma team.

After I was done giving report, the nurse writing everything down looked at my name badge, which has a star of life with wings flanking it, the symbol for air EMS, my name with my title, RN, CFRN.

"What does CFRN stand for?" she asked. Even many hospital nurses don't know what it means.

"Certified Flight Registered Nurse," I told her without thinking about it. It was not an uncommon question.

I had her sign my chart, I wrote the time on it and ripped off a copy and gave it to her. I glanced around to see Brian had all of our equipment and we left.

"Well, that's a save," I said to Brian as we headed back to the elevator. He nodded vacantly acknowledging my usual comment after a call.

Brian is a few years younger than I am, which, unfortunately, does not make him very young. This is not a business with a lot of very young people in it. I'd have to say the common age for most of the medical crews is in their thirties and forties. To be in flight, you have to obtain your degree or certification as a registered nurse or a paramedic. Then you have to put in three years or more working in that field before you can even apply for a flight position. There are some who have the vision and the drive and get into it in their mid-twenties. But more commonly, they're generally in their thirties when they start and well-seasoned. Then, if they last, they typically stay in it for a few years. I started when I was thirty-six and have been doing it ever since. As for the pilots, the same thing applies. They range in age from early thirties up to retirement age. They have to obtain a license for a helicopter and have at least 3,000 hours of flight time just to apply for medical transport. That's a long time, considering that most pilots average about 300 to 500 hours of flight time a year. More if they're lucky, or are past military, or worked for a tour company.

ANOTHER DAY

Brian had been a paramedic for well over ten years. He was recently divorced, with custody of his daughter, who was four years old. He lived in the small town of Sierra Vista, which is south of Tucson. At five feet seven inches, he was stocky and muscular. Short light brown hair and sporting a goatee, he was very quiet and reserved. Except when it comes to his daughter, which is the only priority in his life.

Bud was ahead of us, walking to the elevator, Brian was next to me. I caught out of the side of my eye him suddenly stop and turn around. Curious, I glanced back to see what distracted him. I followed his gaze down the hall and then spotted one stunningly gorgeous nurse standing at the desk in the middle of the emergency department. He took a moment then turned back around and just walked on without a word but with the slightest nodding as he walked. He looked at me silently with a slight grin as he passed by. I couldn't help smiling. I concurred with his assessment. Bud was completely oblivious.

Within minutes we were back at the helicopter. The sky to the east was getting light. Once we reached altitude you could just make out a slight glow of orange on the horizon. When we landed back at the base, however, it was still pretty dark and quiet around the airport. Within an hour, this place would start bustling with morning people and student pilots, all trying to get some flight time in before the day got unbearably hot.

We had a couple hours before the next crew would be here. Brian got the helicopter back to ready-to-go status while I went in and faxed the paperwork to the billing office back at our headquarters. Bud finished some of his own paperwork before Matt Uhl came in to relieve him.

Matt wasn't one of our regular base pilots. His normal base was Native 1 at Williams-Gateway Airport, where we all started. Occasionally, however, he'd come up to do some overtime when one of our pilots wanted time off. I knew Matt really well and liked him. You couldn't help it. Matt was one of the youngest of the first four pilots in the program when it started. He was in his early thirties. Matt had been flying for one of the TV news channels in town. Coffey, the director of the rotor-wing component of NAAA, had hired him. How Coffey knew him, I didn't know. The aviation industry is a pretty close-knit group, especially the helicopter pilots that fly in the Phoenix area. Most pilots know each other, if only by reputation or having talked to each other on the radio.

Even though this was Matt's first "aeromedical" pilot job, he was a very accomplished pilot. Perfect for this type of work; experienced, very easy going, eager to learn, quick to pick up, and extremely non-judgmental. Matt had a mild manner that made him easy with a soft voice. At first, I didn't think he even knew any curse words. He never talked about women or commented on the really cute ones, like most guys would. To him, there was only his wife. His eyes never "window shopped." Most people do, it's a natural thing, but not with him. He was what most people would consider very straight-laced, with a character that was pure. But he had a great sense of humor. Coffey used to call him "Mrs. Uhl's little boy." A title that kind of summed him up and it also stuck, at least with the first crews that were with Native American Air Ambulance at that time.

When NAAA first started up, there was a limited crew that flew on the rotor-wing. There were only four pilots; Coffey, Rick, Troy, and Matt Uhl. So, the medical teams got to know them pretty well in the first few months before Native 2 was started. Then there were four more pilots added. All of them hand-picked by Coffey. The one thing you never had to worry about was that if Coffey picked the pilot, they were some of the best helicopter aviators in the valley. Matt Uhl was certainly no exception to that rule.

About two months after we started, I was on shift with Matt when we got a call. After checking to see if we were ready in the back, instead of saying, "I'm firing up" or "Starting up" or "Coming hot" as was usual, Matt said something else: "I'm going to crank the *shit* out of it."

It was so unexpected and uncharacteristic coming from him, it caught me completely by surprise. I was kind of shocked, but it was hilarious. Mostly because it came out of the mouth of Mrs. Uhl's little boy. That line stuck with me and would come to be the line that I associated with Matt when he was at his finest. Just being on shift with him, you knew you were going to have a good time.

My sleeping room was near the front door to the quarters, which meant you could hear when someone came in. Once I heard the new crew come in, I got up and collected my stuff to go home. I came out and heard Matt address me very formally, "Good morning, Mister Bell." As a gentleman would. I was pleased to see him and spent a good bit of time chatting and catching up.

Once the narcotic box was checked off with the new crew and everyone was done with their shift brief and cordial morning banter, Brian and I left to go home. Another shift down, another dollar made, and another life saved. Yup, that's what we do. We save lives. Well, that is not really what I am thinking. I'm thinking more along the lines of, "Hell, yeah, time to go! I got things to do." The one call we had could have just as easily been taken in by ambulance due to the extent of his injuries, but we were called due to the distance and the possibilities of more severe injuries. But it was a call and we chocked it up on our roster. I got into my little red Corvette and drove home to my wife, who had just come back from taking the kids to school. Now my home life started. It was about eight o'clock in the morning and a whole different life was now underway.

Chapter 2
DON'T LOSE YOUR HEAD

I was sitting on the couch in the living area talking to Bob, one of the medics assigned to this base. Like me, he was an "old-timer." One of the original employees when NAAA first started, Bob had seen it all and had been a part of it all and in some cases, he started a lot of it. Bob had a unique sense of humor about him. He had all the charm of a backwoods, deep home-spun redneck cowboy to him, without any of the usual prejudices. This guy loved his hats and boots and sported a long hanging mustache. A full hanging mustache is traditional with old firefighters. Not only was he a paramedic, he was also a firefighter. After spending time with the crews, you find out things most people don't know. Like the fact that while in the Army, Bob had been a sharp-shooter sniper. Not what you'd expect from this very laidback, southern twang speaking humorous hillbilly.

Bob was a verbal prankster. He would tell people, "Be sure you don't spell my name backwards." Bob would also use words to label things that were not in the Webster dictionary. He'd call things "doohickeys," "thing-a-ma-bobs," "chilliwhoppers," "flicky-dos," and all sorts of other things. You might hear him say something like, "If you don't get that flicker-job stuck into that chilliwhopper, we ain't ever gettin' this dang thing going." Yet everybody knew exactly what he was talking about and what they needed to do. It was a language that everyone could understand but nobody else could speak.

In our quarters, the living area with the TV in it was separated from the pilot's office by a wall and door. Don, the pilot this evening and our aviation manager for this base, was leaning on the threshold into the pilot's office, joining the conversation. Don had a striking resemblance to the politician Joe Lieberman, but don't ever tell him that. I mentioned it one time, totally unaware of his politics, and received a very cold gaze thrown at me. Don was all business. A man who went by the book. As manager, he used the book to his advantage to get what he wanted. Smart.

Bob and I had been here since the morning but Don had just come on about an hour-and-a-half before. The medical crew worked twenty-four-hour shifts. The pilots were mandated to just twelve-hour shifts. With all of Don's beginning of the shift duties and pre-flight out the of the way, he was into killing some time until we got a call or bedtime, which ever came first. We were all comfortable, chatting, with the TV halfway through some movie that we were not really paying any attention to.

The Nextel radio toned out with a "be-leep, be-leep." We knew this was a call. At the beginning of every pilot shift change, the Nextel would go off with the dispatcher checking in for pilot, crew, aircraft readiness, and weather status. That had already been done. So, we knew this was for a call. Don retreated back into the office to get the phone while Bob and I pried ourselves out of our comfortable positions.

"I'd been wantin' to see that dang movie, too," Bob joked on the way to his room to change into his flightsuit.

Within thirty seconds, we had our flightsuits donned and boots on and were on our way out. Being the last one out, I checked that we had the keys and locked up.

In our business, we did two types of calls: hospital transfers, where you take a patient from one hospital to another, also known as an interfacility call, and scene calls, where you actually go to the scene of a serious illness, like a stroke, a heart attack, respiratory distress, or other critical ailment, or a traumatic injury from some kind of accident. In the last few weeks, most of the calls we've had were for hospital transfers. Not to say that they weren't challenging to do also. But scene calls were more engaging. Those were the ones where you had to think a little more out of the box. Plus, you're landing in a different spot every time. That's why the pilots really liked them.

In reality, many scene calls were not that exciting either, despite what most people think. Most of the time, when we got there, the paramedics on scene would already have them pretty much figured out, IVs and oxygen started, bandages and basic treatments already started. Any medications the patient needed immediately, like; breathing treatments, cardiac drugs, or pain medications, have probably already been given also. So, we're left to come in, pick up the patient, and take them to the hospital rapidly.

But every now and then ...

This was another MVA call up on our favorite Interstate 17, just north of Anthem, a small community north of Phoenix. We flew to it in our usual manner, getting the same general scant information from the ground contact. In many instances, the ground crews would have someone designated to handle the landing zone, or LZ, for the aircraft. They wouldn't get involved with patient care or other scene duties. The firefighter in charge of the LZ had very little information about the patient and what had happened. Except for the fact that it was an MVA involving a car and a semi-truck. Well, that's never a good combination. Semi-trucks always win.

Flying over the scene, we could see a semi-truck parked quite a way down from the actual scene where all the commotion was. A black car, looking fairly undamaged, was off to the side toward the median. All the activity was going on between the ambulance and the car. We landed between the car and the semi-truck. It was apparent on our approach that the patient was just a little way up from the car and the crews were working feverishly on him in the middle of the road.

Walking up to the scene, I took a good look at the car. You can get a lot of information from the condition of the vehicle. Sometimes it was hard to look at. Typically, with this kind of damage, the inside of the passenger's compartment looked like a bloody war zone. Not in this case. Except for the front windshield being smashed in, this car looked pretty clean.

Coming up to the treatment area, Bob jumped down and started assisting the rest of the crew getting the patient immobilized on a backboard, with neck collar and head block on. I went to the firefighter writing the report as I knew he would have the information I needed.

This was a young male, late twenties, driver of the black car that was wearing his seatbelt. From what he could gather, the semi-truck's left front wheel had blown out. Not the tire, the whole damn wheel. Huge metal debris had exploded all over the roadway, right beside this guy in the black car. When they arrived on the scene, they found the victim unresponsive but breathing, sort of, still sitting in his seat. No obvious signs of bleeding anywhere in the car or on him and no obvious signs of trauma. Just a huge chuck of some metal piece sitting beside him on the seat.

"We figure he had a head trauma," the firefighter said. "So, we pulled him out, keeping his spine immobilized. That's about all we got. I don't even have a name."

"You didn't see any injuries?"

"Nope, just an abrasion to his right cheek. But that's it." He shrugged.

I stepped over to the flurry of activity. Bob and another paramedic were both starting an IV on each arm. Another medic was hooking the patient up on the monitor. I started doing an assessment of what I could get to. With all the other people working on him, it was difficult to squeeze in. The first thing I confirmed was that he was breathing. Not too fast and not too slow, not particularly deep but breathing. Not making any weird gurgling sounds or anything to indicate an airway problem. But I still had an uneasy feeling about his breathing. My gut was telling me it just wasn't right. No injuries to the head except for the aforementioned abrasion to the right cheek. Pretty angry looking abrasion, very severe skin damage with some blood oozing but no laceration noted. Jaw appeared to be intact. No bleeding noted from the nose or ears, which would be an indication of skull fracture. I got down awfully close to his face to check his pupils and as I'm checking him out I don't smell any odor of alcohol. His pupils were dilated and slow to react, but they did contract a little. That meant that there was still some brain activity going on. That's encouraging.

I glanced at the monitor and see his EKG showing a normal heartbeat, a little slow at about eighty, but normal. I would expect a little higher rate with his body being traumatized. The automatic blood pressure was still running. I started listening to his lungs and heart sounds. All there, nothing abnormal. I felt his chest and abdomen for anything out of the ordinary like fractures, crunches of air under the skin, or unusual warmth like bleeding in the abdomen or elsewhere. Nothing. I looked at the arms with IVs running now, nothing abnormal. I moved down to the legs quickly and felt them and the pelvis. Everything seemed fine. What's going on? Had to be a head injury. But how bad? Was he going to come around in a minute, wondering what the hell was going on? Or was he bleeding into the brain and going to crash on us any second now? My concerns grew and I was starting to get more focused on a patient that could get really serious very quickly. A Glasgow Coma Scale, or GCS, is an indication of brain function. This patient's GCS was a three. That's as bad as you can score. A dead person scores a three, literally. Normal people score a fifteen.

Blood pressure finally came up on the monitor, 101/42. That was low. I spent less than a minute getting all this information doing the assessment. The trauma unit was about twelve minutes from here. We needed to go, but he really needed a secured airway. He needed to be intubated. Bob was already getting intubation equipment out and ready.

"He's crashing!"

I was not sure who said it, but they weren't wrong. I looked at the monitor, and his heartbeats were quickly slowing down, 48-36-32-24. Yup, he was crashing. We all got ready to code. To "code" is a euphemism used by medical personnel to signify a cardiac resuscitation. That's when you see everyone on TV doing CPR, screaming, "Clear!" defibrillating patients, and shoving breathing tubes down patient's throats. It's high drama. It's important not to lose your head in these tense situations. It's scary and exciting all at the same time. I flashback to a book I once read early in my nursing career: "Remember, it's the patient's emergency, not yours."

"Let's get him an amp of Atropine in now," I said calmly. Atropine is a drug that should speed the heart rate up. The on-scene paramedic grabbed his drug box and pulled the drug. On a normal scene, with paramedics already on site, we didn't bring our big drug box with us. It was cumbersome and besides they already had one on-scene. However, I always brought my little drug box that had drugs ground crews don't carry.

I looked at Bob. "We're going to need to intubate this guy now." Indicating we needed to put a breathing tube down his throat into his lungs.

"All ready. Let's do it!" Bob handed a mask and ambu-bag to start giving artificial respirations, as the guy's respirations are becoming very slow and erratic.

There are two things you should never let happen if someone has a head injury, or bleeding in the brain. One, never let their blood pressure drop. Two, don't let their oxygen saturation drop. We had to keep his pressure up and keep him oxygenated.

"Get another pressure," I said, meaning to push the button for another automatic blood pressure.

"Do we have an OPA," I asked.

Bob tossed up an oral pharyngeal airway. "Here's that little curved doohickey to put in his mouth."

I rotated it in, placed the mask on his face, and started squeezing the ambu-bag, "bagging" the patient to get his oxygen concentration back up and steady. I noticed on the monitor that the heartbeats were coming back up after the Atropine was given, 46, 56, 72, 84. That was encouraging. That worked. The blood pressure popped up on the monitor, 108/52. That was a plus. But he still wasn't breathing much on his own. In this case, there was no need to give any drugs to make the intubation tolerable for the patient. This would be a "crash airway." In other words, he was so unresponsive and limp that there wasn't going to be any problem pushing a tube down his throat. Except for the fact that I couldn't bend his neck back to make visualizing the vocal cords easier. Couldn't afford to manipulate his neck at all. It had to remain in-line and stable, in case of a neck fracture.

Bob handed me the scope to look down the man's throat. With all the equipment in hand and ready, I put the laryngoscope in his mouth and looked down his gullet. With a little help from Bob pushing in on his throat to manipulate his vocal cords into a better position for me to see, I was able to at least get the landmarks I needed to identify where I was in his throat. I could make out the area I needed to be in. I couldn't clearly see the vocal cords at this angle, but I knew where they *should* be and I guided the tube to that space. Semi-blind to where the tube needed to go, I positioned the tube where I thought it should go and pushed it in. It felt and looked right. I inflated the balloon on the end of the endotracheal tube that holds it in place and listened to his chest. I had the paramedic squeeze the bag that was now attached to the breathing tube while I listened, first over the stomach to make sure it didn't go straight down the esophagus. That would mean I passed by the trachea going into his lungs and inadvertently went down the passage to his stomach. All I would do then was blow his stomach up like a balloon. Then I listened over the lung areas. No sounds in the stomach, good breath sounds in both the right and left lung areas. I put a CO_2 detector device on the tube just to confirm proper placement in the lungs, and it confirms that it was in the right spot by changing colors when exhaled CO_2 from the lungs hit it. I was in the right spot. I'd take that. We started bagging the patient at a smooth rate to keep his oxygen level up.

I looked at the monitor to see if his oxygen saturation was good, which it was, but noticed abnormal heartbeats popping up and becoming more frequent as I was looking.

"Can we get him a shot of Amiodarone?" I asked one of the paramedics. A drug that should stop the abnormal heartbeats. I can ask, I can even strongly suggest, but I should never demand a paramedic what to do. It was a quick way to become unpopular. The paramedic reached into his drug box, retrieved the drug and gave it.

I watched the monitor for a moment while a couple of the fire guys secured the intubation tube. I pushed the button for another automatic blood pressure. As it was running, I noticed the heart rate start to slow again. The blood pressure came back, 92/42. He was going back down. Damn!

"Let's give him an amp of Epinephrine," I indicated to the paramedic. Epinephrine is another name for Adrenaline. "And, let's get ready to do CPR."

With that, a firefighter positioned himself beside the patient, ready to start doing compressions as soon as directed.

I watched the paramedic bagging the patient. Not unusual, he was bagging just a little too fast. When the situation gets stressful, it's normal to squeeze the bag pretty quickly. Time gets obscured easily. "A little slower," I suggested. He understood. We didn't want to hyperventilate this patient. That could be just as bad as not giving him enough breaths. It's very easy to start bagging a patient at the same rate at which you, yourself, are breathing.

Looking at the monitor, I noticed that the Epinephrine had done its job well. The heart rate was back up and his blood pressure was climbing. I took a good look at everything, the intubation tube was well secured, the patient was being bagged at a steady, proper rate, his vital signs were about the best we were going to get for now. It was time to move. Everybody got a corner of the backboard and with the paramedic who was bagging counting to three, everyone lifted. I stayed hands-free so I could stand back and see all sides and everything going on. I wanted to make sure we didn't have a tubing lying somewhere it could get stepped on, or something hanging that could get snagged and pull something out that's vital while carrying him and putting him in the helicopter. With everybody working in unison, we made our way to the aircraft.

Don, sitting in the pilot's seat, could see everything going on and coming his way. When we got close, I ran ahead to open the door and prepare the inside for the coming patient.

I shouted to Don over the din of the engine. "Twentyish-year-old male, 175 pounds, unresponsive, intubated, going to JCL Trauma, cold off-load right now!" Everything he needed to know to get this party started. He relayed the information to dispatch to patch over to the hospital for a heads up.

The team arrived with the patient, slid him onto the stretcher inside the aircraft, and left. I continued to bag the patient until Bob could get in and take over. Under the loud thumping of the rotor blades the fire captain put his hand on my shoulder and shouted, "Anything you need? Got everything?"

I nodded my head and thanked him. "Good work, you guys."

He patted my shoulder, ducked, and hurried out from under the blades. Bob was already in the aircraft getting IV bags hung, the monitor secured and pulling out the ventilator. When everything was ready, he took over bagging the patient as I closed and secured the door. I took a quick glance around to make sure everything was ready for our departure and then scurried around and climbed in. As soon as I let Don know we were good, he pulled pitch and we were off.

I started setting up the ventilator to take over the respirations for this patient. I knew this guy was going to keep us busy on the way into the hospital and I wanted both Bob's and my hands free. And the patient didn't disappoint. Shortly after we lifted his blood pressure started to tank. His heart rate remained the same, however. Very common for someone with a brain or spinal cord injury.

For most people, when their blood pressure drops, their heart rate rises. It's a normal response. Unless that's the reason the blood pressure was dropping, because their heart rate was dropping. But when the cause is neurogenic in nature, in other words, caused by an injury to the brain or spinal column, the heart doesn't respond to the decreasing blood pressure. It just stays the same. I didn't find that unusual. It just confirmed to me that this patient had a head injury. Or, neck. A neck injury was still in the running for possible causes too. But, right now, I didn't really care what the cause was; I just knew I needed to do something. So, I started a vasopressor drug, which increases blood pressure by making blood vessels squeeze down tighter. One of the two things you don't want to happen when the brain is injured is the blood pressure to get too low. With me programming the IV pump and Bob priming the IV tubing, we got the vasopressive medication IV drip started pretty quickly. Good results, the blood pressure stabilized. We were able to maintain good oxygenation and good blood pressure all the way in to the trauma center.

Without missing a beat, Don deftly dropped Little Girl

right onto the helipad like coming into a hot LZ. The patient seemed reasonably stable for the moment, so we went through the routine of a cold off-load, which is shutting down the helicopter. Within minutes we were in the trauma room, and the trauma team jumped into action. After a quick trauma assessment, he was whisked out of the trauma room to CT for a scan of the head. No wasting time here. Shit, I barely finished my report and got a signature before they were headed out. In fact, I had to step aside to let them push the gurney past. I helped Bob pick up our stuff and wipe it down.

"I thought that furry wombat was a goner there for a bit," Bob commented.

"Yeah, he's not doing so good," I replied. "But that's a save in my book."

"Yes sir. Yup. That's a save for sure."

"What the hell, though," I exclaimed, thinking about all the lack of injuries and indications. "What the hell happened?"

"I heard one of the fire guys say a piece of brake lining from the semi came through the window."

"Brake lining?" I reflected. "That's what left that gnarly abrasion on his jaw. I'm surprised he wasn't gushing blood. What are the odds in that?"

"Hey, if God's going to get ya," Bob said, "he's going to get ya."

I thought about that for a moment. "Yeah, that's why I don't get it when people kill in the name of God. If God wants you dead, God doesn't need any help from people."

"That's for sure," Bob replied.

Before we left, we heard them call a code blue in CT. Knowing that our patient was in there we sort of hung out, curious to learn the outcome. We got word that the patient expired and was pronounced dead in CT. That quieted our mood considerably. Having heard enough, we decided to go on and leave.

Now I was left wondering whether we did everything right! Did I do something wrong? Did I not do something that I should have? This chart would certainly be scrutinized by several people, all with their own opinions. No one is harder on you than yourself when it comes to second guessing. What could I have done differently?

On the way to the elevators the trauma doctor came up to us. "Hey, you guys want to see this?" he asked.

"Yeah," I said, curiously. Not knowing exactly what I was agreeing to see.

We followed him into the CAT scan room, where the body of our poor man was draped with a sheet on the table that slides you into the machine. All around the floor were wrappers and boxes of the failed, furious efforts of the trauma team's attempt to save this patient. We continued to follow him back into the control room with the computer screens. He had the tech pull up the films they acquired just before the man died. The doctor pointed at an area on the film just below his skull.

"You see that?" he said.

I'm not an expert at reading CT scans, I'll be the first to admit that, but when something is obvious, it stands out to anyone. Even to a novice radiologist like myself. I've seen hundreds of CT scans. I've been taught how to read spinal cord injuries from numerous courses I've taken through the years. Many classes and clinical rotations that have been mandated for certifications to maintain my job. I have never seen one quite this obvious even at a quick glance. Where the spinal column attaches to the bottom of the skull, there was a gap of almost two inches. Not only was there a two-inch gap that shouldn't be there, it was displaced about an inch behind where it should be. This was known as an internal decapitation. This man had been decapitated from the piece of brake lining coming through his windshield.

"It's a wonder that you guys got him this far," the doctor said, shaking his head. "A wonder."

"Could he have survived this?" I asked. More for my own peace of mind than anything else. Already well aware of the answer.

"No way," he replied. "Like I said, I'm surprised you got him here with a heartbeat."

Bob and I thanked him for confiding the results to us. We don't generally get that privilege. If we would have left, like we normally do, we wouldn't have been privy to this tidbit of information. We were appreciative of that and would be sure to pass it along to the ground crew that was there helping us. They'd want to know too. Like us, they rarely hear the results of their patient's outcomes.

Unaware of it at the time, but an incident very similar to this would come back to haunt me much later.

Chapter 3
AUXILIUM DESUPER

Native 5 was my base. I say that because that's how I felt. I was the first manager of that base. When Richard (Rick) Heape, the owner of NAAA and Coffey, the head of the rotor-wing program, first started talking about putting up the fifth base at Deer Valley Airport, I jumped all over it. I had seniority with the company by this time and after the time I put in and where I lived, Laura, our Chief Flight Nurse, was agreeable to let me transfer to that new base. At the time, I was driving a minimum of an hour to get to the closest base to my house. Sometimes as many as two-and-a-half hours to get to other bases. Deer Valley Airport was less than twenty minutes from my house. When they finally opened it, I went up and was asked to be the first base manager of that location. I eagerly accepted and started a decade-long tenure there.

I came on-board when Native American Air Ambulance was just getting started. Native 1 was our first helicopter in operation. It was out of Williams Gateway Airport, a decommissioned air force base from years ago. Now it was the remanent of an old airport with a very small terminal and many old unused hangars around the periphery. Rick had acquired two of the hangars at the very back of the airport. There he started and housed his new company, starting with two Jetstream aircraft.

These Jetstream aircraft were big. nineteen-passenger airplanes, with twin turbo-prop engines. These were big enough that the FAA mandated two pilots; a captain and a first officer. Much bigger than everyone else was using for aeromedical services in this state. They were laid out with two stretchers on one side and six passenger seats on the other. The Swedish-made Jetstream was originally designed to transport British military personnel out to aircraft carriers. At least that's what I was told. I believed it, too, because every time they touched down on the runway, it felt like the pilots were trying to catch the three-wire. *Bam*! Not much give in that suspension. They were stiff and rough, but they were roomy and tough. You could stand straight up and walk down the aisle. That made it nice for caring for patients, and you could tend to more than one patient at a time.

One of the things Rick said that he wanted to provide was the best. The best aircraft, pilots, medical equipment, and crews. He admittedly didn't know much about the aeromedical industry, at least the medical part, but he did know about aviation. Rick was a seasoned captain with America West Airlines. In fact, this little endeavor was his part-time job and what he dumped his whole retirement funds into. When he started out with this, he would step in personally as captain on many of the flights. Now he just tried to keep up with the growth of the company and making it work.

Because Rick was part Native-American, he received preferential opportunities with contracts with the Native reservations at San Carlos and Whiteriver. That was one of the reasons for him starting this company. He wanted to provide good service to those populations that were not recognized as a priority. However, when it came time for a contract with them, the reservation authorities wanted him to have a rotor-wing component also. So, long story short, he met up with Coffey and teamed up with Omniflight Helicopters, Inc. to handle the helicopters and pilots. Native American Air Ambulance would provide the medical staff and equipment.

With Coffey at the helm of the helicopter component, you had a seasoned aeromedical pilot and manager handling that part as well. We'd call him by his last name, Coffey, as a sense of respect for the head of the rotor program. Just Coffey's presence demanded respect. Coffey knew this industry, after having worked in it for quite a few years. Coffey was tenacious. He wanted this program to work. Partly because it was just his nature to want to be the best at everything he did and partly because he wanted to show up "the other" aeromedical company in town. Coffey was a big, and I mean big, take-no-BS kind of guy. Not to say that he couldn't give BS with the best of them, which he did, and often. It was his personality to work hard and play hard. He was not immune to playing a good joke on you, but when it came to business, that was no joke. He was an All-American man's man. He drove a big pick-up truck, loved skeet shooting, hunting, and his dogs. Over six feet tall and running about 240 pounds, I always wondered how he squeezed his ass into the pilot's seat. The running joke was that Coffey didn't get in the aircraft, he just strapped it on over him. It then became an extension of his own body. He was so good that if you put a quarter on the ground he could land the skid right next to it, touching it. No shit!

He had a tendency to call everyone "Sport." Whether he

was being nice or being sarcastic, it didn't matter. Everyone was just "Sport." "Where ya goin', Sport?" "Hey, Sport, did you do this?" "You wanna get that for me, Sport?" He was in charge. No one ever had to ask, everybody just knew it from the way he carried himself. He was in charge. Don't let that slip your mind, either.

Now, I'm not saying that Coffey was in any way sexist, but that was a persona that he carried around with him. Always quick with a joke, or a jab if he could get one in on you, or a snide remark, like him or not, he was always fun to be around. He was one of those that you, male or female, liked to hate or hated to like. Every woman I knew that knew him, liked him. A lot. Even though my wife used to say, "Matt's a pig," referring to the way he'd talk, I think she secretly had a thing for him.

We didn't have any female helicopter pilots and I remember asking him one time why. He told me he had a test for female pilots.

"I have them put their hands behind their head. Then, I have them walk up to the wall. If their elbows touch first, they don't qualify." Then, he gave me that "do you believe that shit?" look with a half-cocked smile. A couple of years later, he did hire a couple of female pilots with the only standard being quality of piloting skills.

Even though the original crews that started with the company thought about it, we never gave ourselves cool nicknames like "Maverick," "Cool," "Stitch," or anything else like that. We just called everybody by their name. Generally, their first name, unless it was pretty common, then we would use their last name just to differentiate. At one point in the company, if you forgot someone's name you could just call them Mike. You'd have about a 50% chance of being right.

We had so many Mikes. Somewhere along the line, however, Coffey started calling me Cletus. I don't know why or how it started, but before long others were calling me that too. I was never sure if I liked it or not. Still don't know what the hell a Cletus is. Maybe from the old TV show "*Dukes of Hazard*." I don't know.

The first mission done was on July 4, 1997, with the first helicopter we started with, N206AZ. Yup, Little Girl. Only she wasn't known as that yet. When we put up the next helicopter at Chandler Hospital, we got another Bell 206 that looked identical to the first one except it was on high skids. That was when I went to calling them Big Girl and Little Girl. That helicopter was N206MH, but the company designated her as Native 2. Pretty simple to figure that out. When Native 3 was started, Little Girl went up to start that base and they got another helicopter to take over the Native 1 spot. And so it went. Native 4 was our first different type of helicopter, an A-Star B3. The A-Star looks more like a dragonfly. The next base was at Deer Valley Airport, and good ol' Little Girl came over there to start that one up. Truth be told, Little Girl was pretty much the workhorse for the company. She went where she was told and did her job. I loved that bird.

I had an innate sense of pride with Native 5. It was my base and I was the manager. But every team member who'd started the base seemed to have the same sense of ownership with the base as I did. It was our base. We could run it our way. We could do our own thing. As long as it was professional and within NAAA's simple and minimal protocols at the time. I tried to make sure everyone had input in the base. I didn't dictate how I wanted things done. We worked as a group to come up with a way that worked best for us. It was very much a team effort. It kind of had to be, because when we first started, our "quarters" was a twenty-eight-foot motor RV parked on the tarmac. The pilot's office and sleeping quarters were in the back bedroom, and the medical crew stayed in the front living room and kitchen area, where one of us would sleep in the bunk over the driver's cabin and the other would sleep on the fold-out couch bench. Needless to say, before our long-term quarters were built ten months later, it was pretty cozy and we had to get along well with each other.

Trying to bring our team together, I decided to make our own flag. I thought about it for some time. A symbol that would identify us as our own base. Something that we could take to public relation events and show our pride in our base. Something that we could fling in the face of other bases. Yeah, competition is not just between other aeromedical companies. We would be competitive with other bases in our own company.

The company had a logo of an American Indian symbol known as a Zuni. It was a square with three lines coming out from each side, north, south, east, west, like a sunburst. It was on all of our aircraft as a distinguishing visual symbol of Native American Air Ambulance. I put that symbol in the middle of the flag with a "5" in the middle of the Zuni. On top, I had a banner that read "5th Aeromedical Team." On the bottom I had "Auxilium Desuper" printed. Auxilium Desuper was Latin for, "Aid from Above." I thought that was very fitting and noble. I had the flag made. When I got it, I took the flag up to the base and showed the crew. They loved it. Though they had absolutely no idea what it meant. They couldn't even pronounce Auxilium Desuper, much less having any clue what it meant. After I explained the Latin to them, they loved it even more. They warmed up to my little eccentricities pretty well. Native 5 was a great crew. They were my family away from home. They were all great people. We were a team. This wasn't where we worked; this was where we *lived*. We were family. We had pride in our team.

Native 5 went through many transformations through the years, but when we first started, it was our base and it was cool. It was known as the boy's club when we first staffed it. We affectionately called ourselves "The 5 Guys." Unusual for a flight base, all of our staff were male. The company had many female nurses and medics working for them, but our base just worked out to be all guys. Our staff was experienced and easy going. No gossip, no drama, just come in and do your job and go home. A flight nurse who started the base with me was James. Very lean and fit. Quick to laugh, but a very "take-no-shit" kind of guy who was Special Forces in the Army. He knew his job and excelled at it. A great counterpart to me. I knew when I came in after him that everything was going to be checked off and right; ready to go. Up to top standard because that was the way he was trained in the Special Forces.

I asked Brian one day as he was playing a computer game to kill time, what flying with James was like? Did they get along? On occasion, I would fly with James as a partner. Nurses could fly with other nurses when staffing demanded it. But I wanted to know from Brian's point of view how things were going and how I compared to James.

"He's good," Brian said without losing concentration in his game.

Just to continue the conversation, and probably because of a little ego balance, I asked, "Would you rather fly with James or me?"

Brian just remained quiet, concentrating on his game. Aeromedical partners are famous for pushing their partner's buttons. They don't ever want you to start getting an inflated head. They like to keep everyone firmly planted on the ground and never lose that effort to keep trying to be better. In short, they like to pop your balloon. So, his uncharacteristic silence was confusing me. Was he that interested in his game or was he avoiding saying something I might consider disturbing?

Unable to contain myself, I asked, "Why do you like flying with James? How's he different?"

Brian, not looking up from the computer, said, "Uh …" He cleared his throat. "He's smart."

Like I said, a man of few words.

"And he's cool," he added a second later.

I stopped there, figuring further inquiry would not be beneficial to my ego. I decided to walk away and let Brian have peace with his game and not disturb him further. I noticed a sardonic smile come on his face as I turned to leave. Yup, he loved to push that button.

Ah … Native 5, yes, we enjoyed and were proud of our team. We had the feeling that we were "Auxilium Desuper."

Chapter 4
AEROMEDICAL

Helicopter aeromedical work is unique in the realm of response and transport of patients. Primarily due to the mode of transportation used. A helicopter team can simply access locations other forms cannot. Also because of the makeup of the medical professionals employed. Generally, the teams consist of two different disciplines. In our company, we strived to have a paramedic paired with a registered nurse.

Traditionally, a paramedic is trained for first responder emergency procedures. Quickly accessing and assessing patients and their needs. They're hammered in class on the here and now. What do they have to do now before they transport and then get the patient transported to definitive care. Nurses, on the other hand, are trained on what to do once they arrive at a medical facility. What to do now and how to continue care through the long process of recovery. They're hammered in class on a larger array of medications, more advanced treatment devices and theory of long-term care of many diagnosis, from giving birth through to palliative care of the dying.

Two schools of thought looking at patients from different angles. In an industry where we transport emergent patients from a scene and also transport critical patients from one hospital to another hospital for specialized care, it's a good complement. The paramedic is experienced with the recognition and treatment of the emergency patient on scene and how to keep themselves and others safe in what can often be a chaotic mess with many different dangers lurking around. The nurse is experienced on the care of the critical patient on many different medications being infused through IVs and devices, like ventilators, pacemakers, intra-aortic balloon pumps, etcetera. Not to mention the myriad of tubes you can have going in and coming out of one person.

Like some aeromedical nurses, I started as a medic and then obtained my nursing license. I always tried to look at the patient from both sides, concentrating on the angle of the particular situation I was in at the time. However, I always relied on my partner as a resource for us to make the best decisions and give the most efficient and effective care.

When talking about our unique quality, though, it was undoubtedly our vehicle of choice, a helicopter. Unfortunately, in the medical field, having all the knowledge and skills in the world is essentially useless unless you have the right equipment when you need it. I may know exactly what's wrong with you, but short of basic skills like CPR, holding pressure on a bleeding wound or giving you a glass of sugar-water, I really can't do much. I can't even start an IV unless I have an IV needle. We're trained on how to use the equipment and medicines we have with us. When we have that, we're pretty useful. A helicopter is a really useful piece of medical equipment.

Now if you're a cardiologist, out riding horses in the middle of the desert with five of your friends and one of them starts having debilitating chest pain, you may know they're having an acute heart attack. But other than that, you're pretty inadequate. Unless you happen to have a working cell phone. Then we could get the call and fly in to help. *Auxilium Desuper!*

Don, Bob, and I were flying way out east of Black Canyon City, miles from any road, to a place only accessible on horseback. Or, a helicopter. The cardiologist recognized his friend's dire condition and called 911. After explaining the situation to the emergency dispatcher, we were notified and asked to attempt to find and assist the group in the middle of the open desert. He gave the dispatcher an extremely general area to start looking. He had no GPS device available to help pinpoint their location. The area we were heading to was essentially a flat, featureless part of the desert encompassing about fifteen-square-miles of space. The first thing we would have to do was find them.

The two miraculous things working in our favor was the fact that where they were, way out in the middle of nowhere, was exceptionally quiet, you could hear a helicopter from miles away. And, the cardiologist had a fully charged cell phone that was able to get reception where they were.

As the cardiologist was tending to his friend, another in the group was on the phone with our dispatcher, who was relaying the information to us over the radio. The problem with that was there was a significant delay in information. When we arrived around the general area, all of our eyes were looking out straining to find a group of men and horses out in this vast barren landscape. From our position, a horse would be about the size of the lead tip on a pencil held at arm's length, or put another way, about the size of a mesquite tree, which there were a thousand of on the ground out there all over the place.

Dispatch came over the radio, "The reporting party says

that he can hear you. You seem to be south of him." Which would make sense, because we were coming north from Phoenix. At least, I guessed, that meant we hadn't passed them yet.

Dispatch added, "He says, they're about eight miles south of Gopher Springs Road. It's a dirt road that goes some ways out into the desert." Well, that might have been helpful, if we knew where Gopher Springs Road was. There were a few random dirt roads that came out into the desert. But none of us knew any of their names and they were not listed on any of our maps.

"He says he thinks he can see you at about his two-o'clock position," dispatch relayed a few minutes later.

Well, again, that might have been helpful if we knew what direction he was facing.

"He says the group is down in the dry creek bed," dispatch said. We were looking around desperately. From our altitude we could easily see more than five square miles of desert.

"I see about six of them washed out gullies around here," Bob said over the intercom, exacerbated.

These instructions are not unusual coming from a ground contact. Even seasoned firefighters fail to understand what we can see compared to them, it is enormously different. Once, going to a scene in a relatively small mobile home community, we were getting location instructions from the LZ command. The little community had a lot of decorative trees which were great for shading in the summer time but made seeing what was on the ground difficult. He radioed to us, "We're on the east side of the park. There is a blue truck down the street. And right now, I can see you coming in on my three-o'clock position."

From 700 feet off the ground and about four miles out, we could see three parks around the community. Eight blue trucks were sitting on various roads in the area. And without knowing what direction the firefighter was facing, his three-o'clock position meant nothing to us. At night, it is easy to see the flashing lights of the firetruck, but during the day, even a firetruck, can easily get hidden behind some trees. Firetrucks are not that big at 700 feet up. So, we really couldn't fault our unfamiliar helper today.

Dispatch radioed up to us, "He says you're about a mile or so from him and you just passed by." Now that helped a little. But there was a significant distance travelled by the time we got that message. So, when exactly did we pass him and was he on our right side or the left? Regardless, we turned around slowly looking for any dry riverbeds within about two miles from us. That narrowed it down to about three possible directions to shoot for. We started heading to a wash about a mile or so to the southwest of us.

"He says, you're going the wrong way," dispatch alerted us. Okay, well that rules out one possibility. However, that was still pretty vague, which part was the wrong way? So, Don turned the bird back around slowly. Through trial and error and after about another ten minutes, I heard Bob announce, "Tally-ho. I got those willy wombats about ten o'clock and one mile."

After a few seconds, Don confirmed, "Okay, got em." It was hard to see the group because they were in a deep gulley. Only a half a mile away they were hidden below the rim of the chasm. The man on the phone was standing on the ground above the ravine.

Don was unable to land down in the ravine by the patient because of the nature of the riverbed. Not to mention, that unlike humans, horses don't think helicopters are fascinating. It scares the hell out of them and they'll bolt. So, he had no option but to land on the flat desert close to the edge of the rift. That made the trip to the patient about two-hundred yards down the sides of this small canyon over soft dirt and rocks. Everything had to come with us; drug box, monitor, trauma bag, oxygen tank, and the stretcher.

Coming up to the group, the cardiologist introduced himself and made it clear that he was a doctor. He could come in handy but he could also present a problem. In a hospital, with a cardiac catherization lab close by, he would be a great asset but out here I wasn't sure if he would know how to put in an IV or even prime the IV tubing. There was only so much that could be done in the middle of the desert and we were pretty good at doing that on our own. Right now, he was really just a bystander.

Just looking at the man sitting there, I knew this person was in trouble. The look on his face was awfully revealing. He looked distressed, pasty, very clammy with gasping respirations and complaining of severe chest pain radiating to his left shoulder. I immediately put him on oxygen and set up to insert an IV, while Bob was attaching the monitor and blood pressure cuff. While doing all this, I was asking the man some information, like his name, age, medical history and such. I learned his name was Ron, he was fifty-five years old and he had no medical history to speak of.

We ran a quick EKG and looked at it. It didn't take a cardiologist to see this man was having a full-blown heart attack. Without getting into much detail, the waveform that I was looking at is known as "tombstone ST elevations." Well, the name says it all. It's bad. I handed the strip to the doctor while I went on and started an IV and Bob gave him aspirin and then a nitroglycerin under the tongue. As soon as the IV was running, I went on and gave him some morphine also. Without wasting any time, we got him onto the stretcher with the help of his friends. There was no way I was going to let this man try to walk to the aircraft.

We were going to need to carry Ron out of the ravine and up to the aircraft with the help of his friends. One of his friends was about 150 pounds, Ira, the cardiologist, was about 180 pounds, the other two were about 190 to 200 pounds. Ron, of course, was 258 pounds. It always seemed to be the heaviest one that has the problem. One of the men was going to stay back and tend to the horses. I gave Ron another nitroglycerine pill under the tongue before we started out. All of the medication we had given him was starting to help the pain and make him look a little more relieved.

With Ron in a reclined position on the stretcher, in unison we picked him up and started heading for the helicopter. Four of his friends were helping, two at the foot and two on either side of the stretcher, Bob was on a top corner of the stretcher and carrying the trauma bag, I'm on the other top corner of the stretcher and carrying the monitor. Because of the pronounced slope of the sides of the ravine right here, we had to make our way down a good bit farther than the way we came down to carry him up. Extending the distance by another one-hundred yards. Once we got on top of the edge, back on flat land heading to the aircraft I started looking longingly at the oxygen mask on Ron's face. I was thinking, this would probably be a good time to stop this nasty habit of smoking.

Once we loaded Ron onto the helicopter, I reassessed him. He had markedly improved but still needed to get to a cardiac care center quickly. Ira briefly inquired if he could accompany us and was surprisingly understandable when we had to deny him because we didn't have the room. I thanked everyone for their help and they reciprocated with gratitude for helping their friend. After getting Ron settled in the aircraft and with the success of the previous medications, I started to run nitroglycerine at a continuous controlled rate through the IV.

Without further incident, we arrived at the closest cardiac care center in eighteen minutes. We didn't even stop in the emergency department, we were met at the helipad by a security guard and a nurse from the cardiac cath lab who guided us directly into that room. The cath lab team were all there standing by when we walked in. Transfer of care was quick and unhampered and we were out.

"Well, that's a save," I remarked heading out.

Bob nodded, smiling. "Yeah, that's what it's all about, right there."

Chapter 5
NURSING

I started out my healthcare career in the Army as a medic in 1976 and then I became a nurse in 1982. I started as an LVN, Licensed Vocational Nurse. The same as an LPN in some states, Licensed Practical Nurse. In Texas, they were known as LVNs. An LVN is a lower degree than an RN. You can apply for that license after one year of schooling and much less clinical practice time. When I got out of the Army as a medic, my DD214 stated that I was the equivalent of a Practical Nurse. Yeah, well, states and hospitals don't see it that way. You have to go through an accredited nursing program of some kind to be a nurse working in a hospital anywhere. After the Army, I started working at Huntsville Memorial Hospital as an operating room orderly. Yes, in those days they were still called orderlies and they still had them. I was going to college at the same time for pre-med. I wanted to be a doctor.

The girl I was dating got pregnant and we decided to get married. Anyway, I had to work full-time instead of going to college full-time. The hospital I was working at offered an LVN program. I took that instead, so I could be making enough money to care for a family in a year instead of ten to fourteen years to become an MD. I ended up marrying her, having a son, and becoming an LVN.

Because I excelled so well in nursing school, and possibly because I knew everyone in the hospital from working there, I was immediately placed in the Intensive Care Unit as a full-time nurse right out of school working night shift. I did everything that any of the RNs did as far as caring for the patient, from hanging blood, pushing IV cardiac medications to doing cardiac output readings and interpreting EKG rhythms. About the only thing an LVN could not do was be in charge of the unit. That had to be an RN. It was great experience.

I was also the kind of person who was always learning on my own. I would read everything I could about cardiac care, EKGs, neurological care, trauma care. Anything I could get my hands on that helped me better understand what I was doing, how to care for a critical patient, and what I was responsible for I learned on my own. I was one of the only people at that time to have an Advanced Cardiac Life Support, or ACLS, certificate. Back in those days they weren't required, they were rare. Hell, most people didn't even know where to get one. Nowadays, it's required almost everywhere in any type of hospital setting.

When I first became a nurse, nurses were still wearing white dresses and that white nurse's cap. Male nurses wore white slacks and shirt; we didn't have to wear the hat, thank goodness! At the hospital I started in, there was Victor, an RN, and me, an LVN. We were the only two male nurses in the entire hospital nursing staff. Nursing was not considered a profession for men at that time. Professions at that time were much more gender oriented. There were not many male nurses, just like there were not many police officers or firefighters that were female. Guys were generally not nurses, unless you were one of "those fellas." It was still common for people to think that way. Incidentally, Victor was gay. He may have been flamboyant but he was also phenomenally knowledgeable and gifted, not to mention very humorous. I loved him. Luckily, most nights we worked together. He was my mentor and greatest resource. He taught me an enormous amount about critical care. Sorrowfully, I was crushed when he died of the AIDS virus years later. I miss him greatly.

One patient I had back then was a rare female police officer. I remember her father sitting in the room with her one night when I walked in and him saying, "Well, there you go. That's how the world is changing right before your eyes. My daughter, the cop, being taken care of by a man for a nurse. Tell me things haven't gotten all screwed up." I had to smile, as did his daughter. Yup, times were a changing.

After a few years of working the ICU and ER at Huntsville Hospital, and then as a scrub nurse in the OR at Trinity Hospital, I finished my nursing degree to become an RN.

Matt Uhl was talking to me about nursing one night. It was one of those days without a call and you'd have long conversations with your teammates. Matt was always great to talk with, as he always seemed very interested in the whole medical world as well as you individually. I was telling him that when I started, blood pressure cuffs didn't have Velcro. Blood pressure cuffs were longer than the ones today and wrapped around the arm, almost twice, and were tied off with attached string ties. Then you pumped them up and slowly released the pressure, listening to the pulse with a stethoscope while you watched a gauge. You counted the pulse with your fingers on the wrist, and so on. Today, monitors record the EKG, take the blood pressure automatically, and give you the pulse oximetry reading. Pulse ox readings tell you the oxygen saturation of the blood. That was not even heard of when I started. And all that is done with one machine, the "monitor."

I was telling him some other "old timer" nursing stories when a call came in. Matt answered the radio to get the information of where we were going, then we got ready and headed out.

I came out of the hangar, with Matt beside me going to the helicopter. Bob, close behind us, gathered his stuff and locked up. There was just a slight breeze that was refreshing as we crossed the tarmac. This was a nice time of year in Arizona, when the days are warm and the nights are cool. Shortly, Bob was right behind us catching up quickly.

"What made you want to be a nurse?" Matt asked in passing, a continuation of our previous conversation.

"Well, I'll tell ya," I said, looking straight ahead and maintaining a pragmatic tone in my voice for effect. "I knew early in life that I wanted to be a nurse. I knew right from the start, when I was young, I think I was in the first grade. My mom took me down to the get the bus for school. One of the moms sitting there was breast feeding. Her baby was just suckling away at her breast. So, curiously I asked my mom, "What's she doing." And my mother hesitated for a moment, trying to think how to put it. Then she told me, "Well, the baby's *nursing*." And I thought, hell yeah, *that's* what I want to do for a living. I want to nurse!"

After a second, I looked over to see his reaction. He wasn't there. I glanced back to see Matt and Bob stopped, just standing there in silence, shaking their heads at me.

"What?" I asked.

They continued on to the aircraft, passing by me on either side without a word.

Once they were in front of me, I said, "What! You asked."

Matt did his walk around without reaction. Bob and I climbed into the aircraft and got situated.

Then, Matt climbed in and started grabbing his belt straps and getting comfortable. With our headsets on and as he was finishing flipping switches and checking gauges, he asked, "So, how did that work out for you?"

"Well, it's funny." I said, still serious and straight-faced. "But every time I tried to nurse a cute patient, I was always scolded for not being, you know, professional. It's weird. This is a very contrary profession. Not what I envisioned of nursing for a living."

I went about pulling tape for my leg.

Bob chuckled a little and in his usual strong redneck manner said, "Yup, I could see them not a takin' a shinin' to you nursin' patients."

"I mean, whatcha gonna do?" I added.

Matt put his left hand on the throttle and reached over with his right hand to hit the starter and said, "Well, I know what I'm going to do. I'm going to crank the shit out of it."

Now I allowed a full grin to cross my face. I suspected that these two fully appreciated the total bullshit answer to a reasonable question. It lightened the mood because we had little idea what we were going to, other than a burn patient. Just what we'd find was anyone's guess.

Chapter 6
THE BURN

We were headed to a small village south of Payson. It was essentially a convenience store out in the middle of nowhere with a few travel trailers around. There was a small church, an auto repair shop, and an old 1950s gas station that obviously had ceased operations many years ago. There were a few other little buildings that I am not sure of their function. There was also a small building that served as the quarters for the ambulance crew that was stationed there. It was here as a resource for the quite a few camping areas nearby.

This area is in the foothills. The draw of the area is that it is the first place you'd come to out of Phoenix where the temperature starts to drop to an endurable level. There are much better places; much cooler, much greener, and much closer to water, further on. But it is great for those that wanted to get out with their ATVs.

The little ambulance station was of interest to us because it was better to bring the patient here to wait for the helicopter than have the helicopter try to land around a campsite, or close down a road to land.

A few miles out, we made contact with the ground crew.

They let us know that they were indeed at the helipad in the ambulance, waiting for us. They gave the pilot normal landing instructions and graced us with a little patient information. They were treating a female, thirty-six years old, who had accidentally tripped and fallen forward into a campfire. She was awake and alert with significant burns to the upper chest, arms, neck and face area. Vital signs were normal and she was breathing without problems. They wanted her transported to the burn unit at Maricopa County Medical Center quickly. That was kind of a no brainer to us. She had an IV established and her burns had been cleaned and dressed with wet to dry bandaging during the thirty-five-minute flight time coming up here. She was good to go and you could tell by their tone on the radio that they wanted her loaded and transported immediately. Hot load; fast, quick like a bunny.

That's always a little concerning to me. Their eagerness for us to hurry up. I understand the need to get her to a hospital quickly. That's why we brought the helicopter. Not that it is all that fast. It only cruises at 125 miles per hour. My Corvette goes faster. But the helicopter does it the whole way without slowing down for turns, construction or heavy traffic, and it goes straight to the hospital. Point A to point B.

No, what concerned me was when they feel the need to tell us to hurry up. They already know we're going to move pretty quickly. Why are you telling us to hurry? What do you know that we don't yet? What has you so anxious? *That's* what concerned me. You made it sound like the patient is pretty stable and doing reasonably well. What's causing your voice to rush? Ironically, when they want you to "hurry up," that's probably the time you should actually slow down and take a good look.

I looked at Bob. He looked at me. We both have the same expression and the same response. This had Charlie Foxtrot written all over it. Matt asked if we wanted him to stay hot. Meaning, keep the aircraft running and ready. With both of our heads nodding we told him, "Yup."

As soon as we landed, Bob and I made our way over to the ambulance. Trauma bag and my drug box in hand along with the monitor. The drug box and monitor always came with us but we generally did not take the trauma bag unless we were the first medical team on the scene. Which was pretty rare. Everything that's in our trauma bag will already be at the scene with the other medical unit. This time, however, we just had a feeling. That feeling you acquire after some time doing this.

Murphy's law states: If anything can go wrong, it will go wrong. In this business, Murphy rules. We are forever going to plan B, that's really just the norm. There have been plenty of times we've had to go all the way to plan H. Nothing is ever the same. But many times, things are pretty similar and all you need to do is modify just a little. Some times though, things are wholly different than you expected or were led to believe. That's when you have to become relatively creative quickly.

We hopped into the ambulance as usual, Bob via the back and me in the side door. The smell of burnt hair assaulted us immediately. The air in the ambulance was clear but the smell was so pungent that it almost seemed like the rig was filled with a fog of smoke. Strange how the senses can play with your brain. No one had to tell me this was a burn victim.

While Bob was doing an assessment of the patient, I was getting a report from the medic. Jotting down notes on my tape. As I was getting report, I looked at the lady lying there obviously distressed and just as obviously quite fearful. Her state of alertness was a relief to me in one sense. It was also a little disheartening in another. Burns hurt. There's no other way to put it. Burns hurt. When someone is burned, not only are they in pain, an immense amount of pain, but they're also distressed. Everyone knows that burns are disfiguring, at best, and can be fatal. Maybe not immediately, but eventually. No one passes a significant burn off as insignificant.

When it comes to burns, nobody is racial. It is not good for a white person to look black. It is not good for a black person to look white. This patient was an African American. What skin I could see outside of the dressings was pinkish white. That was not a good thing. Her head looked like the burnt end of a match stick. I don't know how much hair she had before, but now it was just singed to her head. The front part anyway. The back part had been spared slightly but still singed. The tip of her nose was pinkish white where the skin had come off. Her mouth and tongue, which should be pink, were darkened from soot. When she talked the smell of smoke just intensified.

As I was getting report and Bob was doing his assessment, it became clear to me that we were going to have to intubate this woman, whether we liked it or not. Intubation is the insertion of an artificial airway, or tube, down their throat. The last thing you ever want to do is take a person that is perfectly conscious, reasonably stable and able to protect their airway and breathe without problems and intubate them. It goes against everything you feel. But in this case, it was necessary.

It was quite obvious that this lady breathed while she was down in the flame. You could tell that by the singed facial hairs and soot in the airway. When you inhale super-heated gas, or fire itself, you inevitably scorch the delicate membranes of the mouth, bronchial passage and lungs immediately. It's unavoidable. Once you have done that they are compromised and insulted. They are going to react. The way they react to such an insult is to swell and swell significantly. Over a very short period of time, this lady's airway was going to swell so much that it would swell shut and be closed. She could breathe right now without any problem but before long, and I'm talking about fifteen to thirty minutes, she was going to be in one deep shit hole of trouble. There were no ifs, ands or buts, she was going to lose her airway. She had to be intubated. And now! Damn.

Rarely would I come into a scene that would have me tense. I've been around long enough that I pretty much take everything in steady stride. Not much anymore makes me uneasy. This, however, had me concerned because this type of intubation is fraught with pitfalls. Though, on the outside, I'm Mr. Cool. Yeah, no problem, just got this little thing I have to take care of. No big deal. Inside, I'm … shit, shit, shit. By this time, I have done many intubations but every one is new. Patients and circumstances are never the same. In particular, a burn patient with as yet an unidentified amount of swelling.

"She's going to need to be popped and dropped," I told Bob. Loud enough to inform the others of our intentions. Popped and dropped was my little euphemism for popping them with some drugs and dropping an intubation tube down their throat.

"Are you going to intubate her?" the medic blurted out.

Well, so much for trying to be clandestine and not freak out the patient.

"Yes," I replied succinctly.

"Now!" he responded excitedly. This was not a place where the medics get a lot of chances to see such things. At least, not this severe. He just thought we needed to hurry and get her to the burn unit quick. Plus, he wasn't use to seeing a patient sedated and paralyzed on scene.

Unruffled, I looked at him straight in the eyes. "Yes."

I wanted him to understand why I was delaying the transport to do this. "She needs an airway now before she swells up. It's about a thirty-minute flight. You think I should do it before we go?" I asked as a consult. I wanted to bring him into the decision-making process.

I find it is always helpful when you point out the obvious and ask them for their professional opinion. The ground crews are always much more agreeable and helpful when they think they're part of the team and they had a part in making the "educated" decision.

"Yeah, I think that would be best," he replied with eyes a little wider.

Bob didn't even consider what they might have in the ambulance for equipment. He busted out our trauma bag, grabbed the airway kit, and started getting the equipment set up for an intubation. At the same time, I opened the drug box and grabbed what drugs I wanted and drew them up.

Rapid Sequence Induction, or RSI, is a fancy term for the process of giving the right drugs in the right order to put a patient to sleep and paralyzing them to make the intubation process much easier and effective. Even when a patient is heavily sedated they can still bite down when you put something in their mouth. That's why you paralyze them also. The only problem that I ever had about calling it RSI was the "rapid" part. There was really nothing about it that was rapid. It took a little bit of time to draw up the drugs, give them, wait briefly for them to kick in and then proceed to intubate. From the sound of the acronym everybody thinks it should be quick, rapid, but it's not.

I knew from experience that this was going to be a critical intubation. Once we gave her the drugs, she was going to have to be intubated deftly and quickly. Once you give RSI drugs, you, in essence, euthanize the patient. If you can't get them intubated, you just put them to sleep ... forever. The drugs sedate them completely and paralyze them. They cannot breathe even if they try. It's very much like the same drugs they give in a lethal injection for executions, except for the last drug that actually stops the heart.

Because of my concern about the difficulty of this procedure, I wanted to be the one intubating. I knew my skill level and, if anything went wrong, I wanted to know exactly what it was. You weren't going to get many chances here. With the drugs drawn up and laid out, I positioned myself at the head of the stretcher and reviewed my equipment. Bob got in position to inject the drugs at my direction and give me a count while watching the monitor. That was important to the safety and success of the process. This was a procedure that I wanted full confidence in my partner, and with Bob I had that.

I explained to the wide-eyed lady what I was going to do and why. Using her name, Shella, I tried to be calm and comforting and give her a sense of reassurance.

"Shella, the first thing I'm going to give you is a big whopping dose of a narcotic pain-killer. That should help immediately," saying it with a smile to make it seem like the greatest idea ever. "Then, I'm going to follow that with a pretty strong sedative to relax you. You wouldn't mind that right about now, would you?"

She nodded agreeing, with her eyes still wide open and panicked.

Trying to take the edge off, both her and everyone else, I added in a nonchalant manner, "Don't worry, I've done this a few times. You'll be fine."

I looked at Bob, "Go ahead. Give the Morphine."

The narcotic and sedative I was giving was at the highest dose for this size patient. I wanted the highest dose, I didn't care if she stopped breathing. Her breathing status was of no concern. I wanted her comfortable. Besides, I was going to stop her breathing anyway. Her high blood pressure could use a little decrease as well.

You could see when the narcotic started to take effect in her eyes. Still open but not straining. Now Bob was giving the sedative. Slowly, you could see it wash over her. I got the ambu bag and mask ready to start assisting with her breathing, and eventually to take over once the paralytic took effect. Shortly after the paralytic was given, you could see the whole body go limp. That's when things go into high gear. No wasting time here. That was when I had to start using my "ultra-calm" voice. I had Bob hold the mask on her face as I squeezed the bag a few times to get her oxygenation way up. Then, with Bob and I working in prefect synchronization, I slid the blade in her mouth and positioned it. The throat was red and angry and already starting to swell significantly. To my delight, there were the vocal cords staring at me like a wanting vagina. The only thing I could do was take the biggest tube that would fit and slide it in. Perfect. Not a problem. I pulled out the scope and injected air in the balloon at the end of the tube that holds it in place. As I held the tube from moving, Bob put the ambu bag on the end of the tube and squeezed. I listened for breath sounds. After I confirmed equal breath sounds on both sides with a stethoscope and no sounds in the stomach, we secured the tube in place with a "tube tamer." An ingenious device that clamps the tube to a mouth block that is held in place with a strap that goes around the head. After that was done we double checked that everything was secure and all the vital signs on the monitor were going well.

"Bob, you want to go get the ventilator set up in the aircraft while I start another IV?" I looked at Bob with a relieved expression.

With a nod, Bob hopped out of the ambulance to go to the helicopter to set up the vent so we could place it on her as soon as she was loaded. With the help of the ground crew I quickly throw in another very large IV needle. Very large. In fact, when I pulled out a fourteen-gauge needle the EMT standing there almost fainted. A fourteen-gauge needle is the size of a pencil lead.

Just as I was about to insert the needle I saw the EMT stare in disbelief at the paramedic. I knew the paramedic from previous flights up here. He was good and knowledgeable. I worked with him several times, but only briefly just while picking up a patient. He was good people.

"He needs to put in the biggest IV possible," the paramedic told his counterpart in response to his reaction. "Burn patients need a lot of fluids. He'll be able to dump a couple liters in her in no time with that IV." He looked at me for confirmation.

"Yup, absolutely, a butt load of fluids," I nodded to him.

One last thing I wanted to do was change the wet to dry dressings. In the older days, that was common so the bandages didn't stick. Burn centers have since learned that one of the critical factors for burn patients is temperature control. With large burns covered with wet dressings the patient can become cold quickly, even in a warm environment. Not a good thing, especially since I just took away any of her ability to shiver and self-regulate her own temperature.

With the IV inserted and the burns redressed and ready, we started to come out of the ambulance with the patient. Bob had the ventilator set up already and was coming to help. We rolled the patient up to the aircraft, loaded her, hooked her up to the ventilator, and cleared everyone off the pad. Bob went around and got in and started hanging IV bags and getting things situated while I secured the doors. I gave Matt a thumb up as I crossed in front of him and got in.

You could hear Matt already throttling up the aircraft to full power. After a second or two he came over the radio, "All set?"

I looked at Bob then reply, "Yup, good to go."

Off we went to Maricopa Burn Center about thirty-five-minutes away. I pulled out my calculator to do some quick figuring of the "Parkland Formula," a formula which gives you an idea of how much IV fluid this patient was going to need. It is based on her size and the amount of area burned. Burn patients need an immense amount of fluid because of fluid loss from the injured skin. I adjusted her IV flow rate accordingly. That was about it for care. I gave a little more pain and sedation medicine en route to keep her knocked out and comfortable. Breathing was being handled by the ventilator. All she needed now was the burn specialists at Maricopa County. One of the top-rated burn centers in the nation. Their teams were awesome and a pleasure to hand a patient off to. No muss, no fuss, they just took the patient respectfully, gave you a pat on the back, and took over.

After we zipped the patient in the burn center and gave report, we were done with the care of this patient. When I finished my chart and handed the burn team a copy, I came back out to the helicopter. Bob was still cleaning up.

"I'm having a hell of a time gettin' that dang smell out of this chilliwhopper," Bob quipped. Bob, with his been out-on-the-range look, was a hoot with all the different names he had for things and the way he just went about doing things.

"Yeah, I'm thinking that's going to take some time. But," I walked over and patted him on the back. I felt appreciative to have had Bob on this call. Everything went really well. "That's a save."

"Yup, sure nough."

There is a way to estimate the percentage of burn sustained by adding up certain parts of the body. The more area burned the more likely it is to be fatal in the long run. Shella was burned over 40% of her body. What's worse is the area that was burned. It was not like a large patch on her back and legs. She was burned on her neck and face. Very bad places to sustain a burn. Her chance of survival was marginal. Her chance of complete recovery very minimal. If she survived, she was going to have lasting disfigurement to her chest, arms and face. She had a long road ahead of her. Many surgeries, skin grafts, and lots of therapy. Physical and psychological. But if she had any chance to survive and carry on any type of normal life, she was going to get that chance here at Maricopa County Burn Center. Unfortunately, in our job, we probably will never know the outcome. Whether she lives or dies, or how well she does. We were just the transport. We rarely, if ever, get to know any aftermath of the patients we transport. It's just part of the job.

Chapter 7
GO TO THE LIGHT

Jeff was one of our permanent medics at this base. He was redheaded and very lean. What you would expect of someone who was a strict vegetarian and road his bicycle constantly for exercise. He had one of those devices that had rollers in it that you could hook the back tire in and ride your fifteen-speed cycle stationary. He would put it on the landing right outside our quarters on the second floor of the hangar. If you didn't see him in the quarters somewhere, safe bet was he was out there riding away. Not uncommon for him to put thirty or so miles on it in one session.

Jeff was also one of those quiet guys who knows a lot more than you would think. Incredibly knowledgeable, much more than you would expect even from a seasoned medic or nurse. I often wondered why he didn't become a physician's assistant. He had the knowledge and aptitude for it, but he seemed to be perfectly happy being a medic and doing what he was doing. He was good at it, that's for sure. He was another one in the group with a happy and satisfying home life and quite active on his days off. His wife and he were expecting their first child. He was always out exploring different areas of Arizona and totally knowledgeable of the geology. He had a lot of capabilities that came in very handy with this job, like reading maps and coordinates for locations. He was really a convenient guy to have around.

It was getting late and I was lying in my room watching TV. Mike B. was our pilot this evening and was checking out something on the computer, as usual. Jeff was in the kitchen area. It wouldn't be long and he would be turning in for the night. Very health conscious, early to bed, early to rise kind of thing.

It was late in December. In Phoenix, December is a nice month. It doesn't get hot during the day and the nights are cool. Not cold most of the time, just very pleasantly cool. It is the reason we live here and why so many people migrate here during the winter.

I heard the Nextel phone go off in Mike's room. Only this time it was not the alert radio signal, it was an ordinary phone call. That was kind of odd. Curious, I got up and peeked in to eavesdrop. I noticed Jeff was just as interested. It sounded like dispatch was asking Mike questions about a mission.

"Well, let me check," I heard him say. "Where'd you say they thought they were?"

Our curiosity piqued, both Jeff and I made our way into the pilot's office. Mike was looking at one of the various maps pinned on the wall.

"How long you say they've been out there?" Mike asked. After a reply, he added, "And who's asking?"

Jeff and I exchanged glances. Mike looked at us and nodded. Something was coming.

"Yeah, we'll go take a look," Mike said into the phone. "Has this been cleared through Coffey?"

Now Mike looked at us and gave us the recognizable twirling finger in the air. We knew what that meant. Jeff and I darted into our rooms and donned our flightsuits. As I was zipping up my boots, Mike walked by the door on the way out.

"We've got a little search to do."

"Cool," I responded. We were right behind Mike, grabbing our stuff on the way out.

One of the things Coffey and Rick let us do was search missions when requested. Unlike patient transports, search missions were where we would go look for someone lost or stranded somewhere. For them, it was a public relations effort. It was a great way to get the company name in the media in a very positive light. Also, some agencies still had a choice as to which aeromedical company they wanted to use. Most other aeromedical companies didn't do search missions, because it was expensive to operate a helicopter when you probably were not going to be able to bill for it. It was considered a non-revenue flight. If you don't transport a patient, there is no one to bill. But when a fire department would ask for assistance, it was a fine way to gain some points with those particular requesting agencies. Plus, it was a noble thing to do.

We were to look for some hikers lost on the side of Little Granite Mountain west of Prescott. The Prescott fire department knew that NAAA had a helicopter sitting at the hospital and thought they would ask if we could help. So, they called our dispatch office. Native 4, the helicopter based in Prescott, was already on a mission and was not available. Native 5 was available, but it would take us about 25 minutes to get there. They were appreciative and accepted our help.

It may not be cold in Phoenix at night this time of year, but

Prescott is another matter. They are higher up in elevation. It gets quite chilly up there at night, especially up in the mountains. These hikers had been out all day and had become lost trying to get back down the mountain. They had used a cell phone to call for assistance but didn't get much information out before it lost power and went dead. It was enough information, though, for the fire department to recognize that they were in trouble and needed help. The fire department said they thought they might have even heard that one of the hikers was injured, but they could not be sure. Regardless, it was getting very cold where they were and expected to get below freezing on the mountain tonight. This could become serious.

Mike was up for the challenge. Being a retired Maricopa County Sheriff Officer, search and rescue missions were right in his wheelhouse. Plus, being an old biker from the '70s, he was up to a little adventure. I was just glad I didn't have to write a report. We got to go for a helicopter ride without paperwork … score!

When we got there, the fire department and volunteers were at the base of the mountain, making their way up the various trails and calling out, trying to locate the hikers. One of the fire guys had a Garmin GPS device and radioed coordinates to their location. Mike handed Jeff the map while he input the information into the aircraft. Within minutes, Jeff's mapping skills paid off and he had located the approximate scene. That's where we headed to. This was a treat for me because most of the time I'd be focused inside the aircraft either on the patient or on the patient's chart. It was great to just go for a ride where my only duty was to look outside for people.

As we came up on Little Granite Mountain, it was as black as a raven's butt outside. The city lights of Prescott were off to our east and below us was nothing but pitch darkness. This was before anyone was using night-vision goggles. If there was any kind of moon out there, it was keeping well hidden.

Mike was skilled in this type of flying, but he was still extremely cautious. He kept a safe distance from the mountain, especially because it was so hard to discern all the parameters in the dark. Even with the searchlight beaming out, a rock or a tree could suddenly pop out at you if you dare get too close. Not to mention, even at a relative hover, you're still moving deceptively fast. So, Mike was studious to keep a safe distance from any potential obstacles. We were quite appreciative of that. But, that being said, it made people on the ground very small.

As we got close, Mike made contact with the ground team. We could see the dim light of flashlights swiping back and forth in several places. It gave us a general idea where to start. The ground crew gave us their best estimates where they thought the hikers might be, so that was where we headed. Mike got as close as he dared and went alongside the mountain, shining the spotlight across the terrain. When he got well past the area they could be, he pulled away from the mountain, orbited back around, and started another swipe slightly higher. In a somewhat grid pattern. All we were seeing were Pinyon pine and Cottonwood trees, lots of bushes, rocks, cliffs, and a few cacti. At one point, I thought I might have seen a coyote scampering away from the on-coming light. But no people.

We went up higher than we thought they could be and then came back down to start over. We only had so much time that we could do this before we would have to refuel. Generally, that was as long as the company wanted us to continue something like this before returning home. One, because of the cost, but more importantly, we were not available in our service area if an emergency call came out. So, we would stick it out as long as we could.

We came back down and started again. This time we did spot some of the searchers walking up the hill, but no hikers yet. This went on for over forty minutes. We continued until Mike noted that we were getting close to having to terminate the search. Mike was on the radio to the ground crew discussing any further possibilities.

Then, suddenly, Jeff said, "What's that?"

Mike didn't hear him at first. When you're talking on the outside radio, you can't hear the intercom inside.

"What's up?" I asked Jeff. "Whadaya see?"

"I'm not sure," Jeff said softly. "Mike, can you turn around? I'll direct you."

Mike caught it that time and slowed, pivoted, and came back around. "Where at?"

"There. Just about our nine o'clock."

We were all straining to see. I was scanning my eyes back and forth, trying to find what he was looking at. Mike swung the searchlight over to the area.

"Hang on a minute, Mike!" Jeff announced. "Swing the searchlight away for a second."

Mike brought Little Girl to almost a complete stop, hovering. We were all still straining to see. Just about the time we were going to move on, Jeff said, "There!"

What in the hell was he seeing, I wondered?

"There!" Jeff reiterated. "I think I got them. Mike, bring the light back over."

Mike swung the searchlight back over to the general area. He pivoted the aircraft just slightly so he could get a better view of what Jeff wanted.

"Bring it over a little more," Jeff directed him. "Now up a little. A little more. A little more to the left. Up a little. There they are, I got em!"

Sure enough, there were three guys standing by a rock that a girl was sitting on, holding her ankle. Two other girls were standing next to her, obviously cold by the way they were hugging themselves. All of them dressed in shorts and T-shirts. What you would be comfortable wearing on a nice sunny day hiking up a mountain. Not what you wanted to be wearing when it's almost midnight, up in the hills.

Mike got on the radio and directed the ground crews toward the direction of the stranded hikers. One of the teams was only about a quarter mile away from their position, but they were headed in the wrong direction. With the searchlight, Mike was able to lead them right to the spot. We stuck around long enough for them to make contact and ascertain that the girl had a sprained ankle. Everyone was okay and wouldn't need air evacuation. Just in time too, we had just enough fuel to make it back to base without violating our reserve.

Astonished that Jeff was able to find them and curious as to how he did it, I was looking at Jeff. "What did you see?"

"I just saw a faint glow," Jeff said. "The guy was waving his PDA. I caught the glow from the screen."

"His PDA," Mike laughed. "You saw his PDA screen?"

"Yeah," Jeff said, matter-of-factly. "I saw it in his hands, swinging it back and forth, when you hit him with the spotlight."

Jeff. goes about his business, seemingly oblivious to the feat he just pulled off. He saw the glow from a little handheld PDA!

Finally, I said, "Old Hawkeyed Jeff over here, ladies and gentlemen."

"Well," he said with a grin. "Like you say, that's a save." Completely and earnestly modest. That is just the way Jeff was. A tribute to his character.

Chapter 8
THE PHOENIX OPEN

I was sitting in the living area watching Brian play a video game on the TV. Anything to kill some time. Mike was back in the pilot's office on the computer. He was always on the computer. Either checking something out or doing required pilot training online.

It was a Sunday afternoon. I heard the Nextel radio go off in Mike's office. We knew we had a flight. Brian and I both headed in to put on our boots and get ready.

"Scene call!" Mike yelled out from the office.

"Where we going?" I asked Mike.

"The Phoenix Open."

That was a new one. "I didn't know you were into golf, Mike. What's up?"

"Fall injury."

How in the hell do you get a fall injury on a golf course? Someone fall out of their golf cart? Someone trip on a hole and fall? I could see a blunt trauma from getting smacked by a rogue golf ball. Or a golf cart versus pedestrian MVA. But a fall injury?

"Pediatric fall injury," Mike added.

Okay, now this was just getting weird. A kid falling on a golf course? How was a kid on a golf course going to fall bad enough to merit a helicopter response? No, even better question: what's a child doing at a golf tournament in the first place?

We go through our routine and get launched. Off to the Phoenix Open golf tournament. It was not too far from us in Scottsdale, probably a six-minute flight. So, as soon as Mike did all his required notifications to air traffic control, he started to get in touch with the ground crew at the scene.

They were going to have us land on the 18th green of the Phoenix Open. A boy, two years old, fell out of the bleachers about fifteen feet to the ground with a positive loss of consciousness.

As we were coming up on the scene, we were looking for the landing zone they had set up. We spotted it. Right there on the 18th green. Right there. They had actually stopped the golf tournament right there to let the helicopter come in and evacuate the patient. Right there, in front of a thousand spectators and tons of TV cameras.

"Oh jeez," I said. Uncomfortable thinking that we could not be any more on display. Every single thing we did was going to be watched by hundreds of people live and countless more on TV.

Mike brought ol' Little Girl in so smoothly and expertly as you knew he knew he was on film. It was beautiful. Brian and I hopped out, instantly putting on our very best movie star look of concerned emergency medical personnel. We hastily made our way over to where we were directed. As I came up to the scene, yes, right out in front of every Tom, Dick and Harry that was watching golf today, I saw a small child restrained in a

KEDs board. It's a small restraining device designed for young pediatric patients to restrict their movements like we do for adult trauma patients on a long board. Three firefighters were standing there along with a paramedic with a chart. That was the guy I wanted to talk to. Mom was tearfully standing by the paramedic with the clipboard, and two medics were kneeling next to the high-pitched screaming kid trying to calm him down. He might have lost consciousness initially, but he was obviously very conscious now.

"What've we got?" I asked the paramedic with the clipboard. I nod at Mom just in recognition but did not smile. I wanted to look calm, concerned, and professional.

"Two-year-old male, fell from the bleachers fifteen feet to the ground, positive LOC," he replied. "Vital signs stable. LOC was brief. He was awake when we got here. No obvious injuries. Tried to start an IV without success on the first attempt. Want him to go to Phoenix Children's Trauma Center."

Was I hearing this right? We had a kid who fell out of the bleachers and, essentially, got the wind knocked out of him, and we were going to *fly* him to a trauma center? I stayed calm, concerned, and professional.

"Copy that," I said. "Anything else I need to know?"

"No. Do you want us to try and get an IV started?" he asked.

I looked down at the child, briefly, thoughtfully. Still maintaining that calm, concerned, professional look. "No. If it's necessary, we'll get it in flight. Let's move."

I talked to Mom for a moment while Brian finished his assessment and got the child hooked up on the monitor. I informed her that we didn't have room for her to ride with us in this aircraft and reassured her that we would take good care of him. I reminded her to drive carefully to the hospital and not to hurry. The trauma team would be some time with him before they would let her come in anyway, so just be careful.

The truth was, by the time she got there, they would probably be ready to discharge the little guy home.

I thanked the paramedic for the good work and turned to lead the two firefighters that were carrying the boy to the aircraft. Brian was keeping pace beside them with the monitor. Ahead of them, I opened the door and prepared the stretcher for the KEDs board. I keep my headset around my neck while I'm on scene. I put it back on before I got under the spinning rotors. Outside the aircraft, the thing is pretty noisy. But even under the rotor disk, with my headset on, I could hear this kid screaming. Boy, does he have a great set of lungs! Love it. It tells me everything I want to know about the child.

After closing and securing the door, I went around the nose of the aircraft. Just before climbing in, I gave the solitary tail rotor guard a wave and thumb up, as usual. It's all about respect. He's alone, guarding our tail area. I appreciate that. The fact that we were in the middle of the 18th green with hundreds of people watching never entered my mind. We were doing our job, as usual.

Normally, as soon as we take off, a child will get quiet and generally calm down and nod off. A helicopter is probably the best pacifier in the world. Well, it should be, considering it is a million-dollar pacifier. But not with this kid. He whelped and wailed the whole way to the hospital, which did not really bother me at all. Ordinarily, like most people, I don't care to hear someone else's kid crying and wailing. I don't even care to hear my own kids go on like that. But in this case, it didn't bother me. In fact, I was really grateful of it. One, I couldn't really hear him all that well to start with, and two, as long as he was doing that, I knew he was okay. He could be screaming because he was hurting. But that has a certain look about it, it's different. No, this kid was screaming because he'd just been taken away from Mom, put in a huge, noisy, vibrating helicopter with two men he didn't know and strapped down to a board. After waking up in front of a hundred people staring at him, and after having a few firefighters come up to him and strapping him down, and after having someone jabbing a needle in his arm, he really was traumatized. He had just been through a very life-changing event. No, screaming because of physical injury and screaming because of sheer traumatic terror are two different things. This guy was okay. He was traumatized alright, but not physically.

Brian was doing what he could to entertain and pacify the little tyke but to no avail. It was a lost cause. Well, the flight wasn't that long, only a few minutes.

We landed at Phoenix Children's Hospital and unloaded the patient. Walking into the emergency room, we had the usual team waiting for us along with a few other people standing by to watch. Not uncommon in a teaching hospital with doctors and nursing and paramedic students doing their clinical rotations. But there were what seemed to be more than the usual amount of people standing around.

TVs are around everywhere these days. It appeared that a child being flown out of the Phoenix Open was already on the news. I guess everyone was interested in what all the fuss was about.

I gave my report, which was pretty anticlimactic. I finished with my usual, "Any questions?" The room was silent, everyone looked at me, then the kid, then back at me. I knew they wanted more, but I just didn't have it. That was it. I had the nurse sign my chart, gave her the copy, and left.

On the way out, the doctor said, "Did you give the nurse your autograph? Good show."

I nodded vacantly, not really paying any attention to it. Except that it seemed an odd thing to say. Never heard that before.

Mike, Brian, and I walked through the ER and back out to the helipad. "Well, that's a save."

"Yeah, really touch and go there for a while," Brian added sarcastically.

In the Bell 206 helicopter there is a massive post in the middle of the cabin. It severely hinders the pilot from seeing what's going on with the patient. So, Mike asked, seriously, "Was the kid really hurt bad?"

In unison, Brian and I answered, "Nooo." Both of us with a wry grin.

"Well, who's to say?" I continued. "That's the doctor's job."

I paused for a moment, then looked at Mike. "It's possible … but not very likely. Kids bounce. Most likely just got the wind knocked out. But then again, you see people do things that should not hurt them and they get really messed up. And you see people get into things that should really have them screwed up pretty bad, and they walk away without a scratch. You just never know. So, the ground crew was erring on the side of caution. Can't fault them for that."

"Yeah," Brian responded. "But how much of that do you think was for show?"

"You think?" Mike asked.

I shrugged. "I don't know. I would hope not any. I don't think they would call in a helicopter just to impress anyone.

They had a little child that just fell fifteen feet and got knocked out. That falls into the class of a trauma by mechanism. They have a hysterical mother standing right next to them screaming and crying. They wanted to do everything right, so they called in a helicopter. They might have thought differently about it after a bit but we were already on the way. No time to turn back."

"I can see that," Mike said.

We got back in to quarters and as soon as I opened the door, the phone was ringing. I went to answer it.

"Way to go, movie star," I heard the voice on the other end say. "Can I get your autograph?"

I had no idea what he was talking about. I could just barely guess who it was on the other side. "What are you talking about?"

"You definitely owe us some ice cream now, dude."

A common ritual among EMS personnel is that if you're on the TV in the news, or anything else, you owe everyone some ice cream. I figured out who was calling, another nurse from another base. We chatted for a minute, then I heard the call waiting tone. I excused myself from the present call to take the other. Oh boy, how long do I have to field this shit. I answered officially as always. "Hello, Native 5."

"What in the hell were you thinking?" This voice I recognized immediately. It caught me off-guard and concerned me. It was my boss, Rick. He never called someone on something like this.

"What are you talking about?" I answered, startled.

"What were you thinking, waving to the crowd like that? Giving them the thumbs up. What do you think, you're a fucking movie star?"

"What are you talking about." I was genuinely concerned now. He used the "F" word. He didn't do that unless he was pissed.

"You, waving at the crowd. How do you think that makes us look?"

Brian was looking at me now with a perplexed look, shrugging with his palms up in a gesture of "What's going on?" He could hear how loud Rick was on the phone. He could see my expression. He knew something was wrong. I returned a wide-eyed glance that said, "Hell, I don't know."

I thought back on the flight and all I could remember was waving at the firefighter tail-guard as usual before getting in the aircraft. But there was nobody else down there but him. He was completely by himself. I was at a loss. I had no idea what he was talking about.

"All I did was wave at the tail-guard, Rick. Just like I normally do, for guarding the tail. That's all. I swear!" I pleaded.

"Well, that's not what it looked like," Rick shot back.

"I wasn't grand-standing."

"I hope the hell not. That's all we need." The phone call abruptly ended.

"What was that about?" Brian asked.

I stared at the phone for a minute then up at him. "I don't know."

I walked around the counter. "Turn on the damn TV. What the hell is going on?" I said.

It was a little after 4 PM. I'd have to wait until five to see the news. In the meantime, Brian and I had to field a couple more obnoxious calls from colleagues dying to get their digs in. Shortly before five, the call I'd been dreading came through. It was Coffey.

"Way to go, Sport. What were you doing?" Coffey said half sarcastic and half scolding.

I said I didn't know what the hell was going on. I told him everything I knew and everything we did. Coffey knew me better than that. He knew that I wouldn't do something like wave to the crowd.

"It didn't portray the company well," he said counselling. "Situational awareness, Sport. You really need to learn that everyone's watching you all the time. Be careful of that. And if I ever do catch you grand-standing, that'll be all she wrote." His tone softened as we finished the conversation.

Five o'clock. Top story, toddler airlifted from the Phoenix Open. Lead story. Hell, it was even on CNN. National news. And, yes, there I am. Walking around the aircraft to get in. By a fluke, that particular camera angle showed me waving and giving a thumbs up, but it didn't show the solitary tail-guard I was waving to. It showed me waving with about a thousand people behind me all watching, some standing and clapping and cheering, but with my headset on under the rotor blades I couldn't hear a thing. I didn't see them. I had my mind on the mission. I was looking at the lone tail-guard, perfectly innocently. But boy, if it didn't *look* like just what everyone thought. Jeez, something so benign becoming so malignant so quickly. And, of course, the camera doesn't lie. Well, in this case, it lied like a bear rug. Now, I have to suffer for some cameraman's dumb filming angle. Thank you very much.

Thankfully, after checking with the ground crew, and yes, they did check, it was confirmed that all they saw was me waving at the tail-guard. That was going to take some time to hear the last of, if ever. Thanks, kid! Next time keep your butt up in the stands. Better yet, Mom, don't bring your two-year-old to a golf tournament! All this for a simple bounce on the ground.

I love this job. Fucking cameras.

Chapter 9
THE NEWS

Not long before Native 5 started up, I was doing a shift at Native 1. I was sitting with Bob in the green room chatting with some of the other crew members right after suppertime. When NAAA first started, we had two hangars at the back of Williams Gateway Airport. One hangar was used for maintenance and storage. The other hangar housed the quarters for the three crews on duty. Two fixed-wing crews and the rotor-wing medical crew. The green room was the main room in the quarters that the crews would spend time.

It was early fall, so there was still daylight well into the evening. Bob and I both had our radios sitting on the coffee table in front of us. Simultaneously, they both came alive.

"Native 1 scramble, Native 1 scramble for a rollover MVA." That was how dispatch got our attention.

Without hesitation, we stood up, grabbed our radios, and headed out to the aircraft. The fixed-wing pilots were employees of NAAA and, as such, shared the hangar quarters with the medical crews. The rotor-wing pilots were employed by Omniflight and thus had their own separate quarters and office. In essence, it was a block house in front of the hangars on the edge of the tarmac. So, by the time Bob and I got out to Little Girl, Matt Uhl, our pilot tonight, was already halfway through his walk-around inspection.

"Where we going, Matt?" I inquired.

"Oh, it's about twenty miles south of here," he replied without taking his eyes off the helicopter. "Close to Maricopa. Some dirt road off the side of Interstate 10."

"Did he say how bad?" I pressed as I boarded the aircraft.

"Not really. Just said a couple people were ejected from their car when it rolled over. Police are there now with Fire, EMS is on the way." He said as he was getting in the aircraft. In his usual easy manner, he reached over to hit the starter. "Cranking the shit out of it."

This was not unusual; the fire department had arrived before the ambulance and had already determined that someone needed to be flown out. How bad the patient's injuries actually were, was still in question. Whatever the case, we didn't care. This was our job. It was why we were here.

Our company had a public information officer named Michael. He had worked for one of the news networks in town and because of that had some connections. Since we were in the early days of NAAA and we were trying to get known, Rick had hired Michael to assist in that effort. Michael had a radio and pager, so he always knew when we were getting dispatched and for what reason. If he deemed it in any way newsworthy he'd call up the news agencies and give them a heads up. I have to admit, he did get us on TV a lot. As he put it, every second on TV is worth advertising dollars.

Well, Michael must have been doing his magic, because before we even arrived over the scene, there were already TV news choppers covering the story overhead. They kept their distance well above us. They didn't need to be close with the power of their telescopic lenses. They stayed about 1,000 feet above the ground, where we would come in at about 500 feet. All the pilots kept in communication with each other, and Matt knew all of these guys.

During Matt's communications with the ground contact for landing instructions, we also got a little patient information. We were going to get a pediatric patient that was ejected from the rollover. That's how they put it; "a pediatric patient." That didn't sound good.

When we landed, Bob and I donned our reflective vests, grabbed our stuff, and got ready to work. Coming up on the scene, we saw two groups of firefighters and paramedics treating two patients. We were directed to one group treating the child. The scene was a little noisy with the added sound of two news helicopters hovering around overhead. We knew our every move was being filmed. Walking over to that site, I noticed the firefighter with the chart. That was the guy I wanted. Another one was holding up an IV bag and standing by the child, who was already immobilized on a backboard. Two paramedics were kneeling by the kid, taping him down and talking to him. Both groups were calm and working at a methodical pace. Nothing frantic here. Just business as usual.

I walked up to the guy writing on the chart and asked, "What do we got?"

"Two individuals, mother and son, ejected from this rollover," reported the firefighter. "Both negative LOC. You're taking the ten-year-old kid. Name is Jeremiah. He has an obvious broken arm. Vital signs are stable. IV established and he is secured on a long board."

"How's Mom?" I asked.

"She's fine," he replied. "Just complaining of a sore back. No obvious injuries. Palpated the back. Nothing out of place and no complaint of tenderness when palpating the spine. We're going to transport her by ground."

"And the only injuries on the boy is a broken arm?" I confirmed.

"Yeah," he reiterated. "No open wound. Just obviously broken. His left upper arm is deformed. We have an eighteen-gauge IV in his right AC."

"Have you given him anything for pain yet?"

"No, not yet. Figured we could wait for you guys."

"Is he in a lot of pain?"

"Doesn't seem to be," he said, looking over at the boy. "But I'm sure it's hurting."

"Yeah, I would think so," I agreed, looking over also. "No problem. We can fix him up with that."

I finished getting what other information I could, like birth date and past medical history and allergies, which there were none on this ten-year-old kid. Then I moved over to the site where Bob had finished putting him on the monitor. I knelt down next to this kid. This "kid" was about 140 pounds. I looked at Bob and then at the other paramedic kneeling there. This kid was only ten-years-old? I got the same look from both of them.

"Are you hurting, Jeremiah?" I asked the rather large "pediatric" patient lying there.

"My left arm is," he confirmed, in a really mild, composed voice. "Not too bad though."

"Would you like something for it?"

He attempted to nod, when Bob, the paramedic, and the firefighter all quickly told him not to move.

"Try not to move your head," I told him. "Just say your answers. We don't want you to move your head, just in case there's something hurt in your neck. That's why you're strapped down to this board. I know it's uncomfortable, so I'm going to give you something for that and your arm. Okay?"

He attempted to nod again with the same reaction. It's hard to break an instinctive response to an asked question. Especially, when you're trying to be good and help the people helping you. I had to smile a little at his bravery. This was a good kid caught up in a bad situation. I went about drawing up some pain medication.

"How's my mom?" the boy asked.

"She's doing okay," I told him as I injected the pain medicine and added an anti-nausea medication right after it. "She's being taken care of right behind you. She's doing good."

"Is she coming with me?" Jeremiah asked.

"No," I answered. "She's going in by ambulance. But she's going to the same hospital. You'll see her there."

"I'm going in the helicopter?" he asked, half amused and excited, half concerned.

"Yup," I said. Giving him a grin, "You're special."

That brought a grin to his face too.

Just before we took Jeremiah, I dashed over to where the crew was taking care of the mother. I figured she would be concerned about her boy, so I wanted to let her know how he was doing, what we were doing and tell her not to worry, he was fine. She expressed her appreciation and I went back.

Everyone ready, we picked Jeremiah up and carried him to the waiting helicopter. There we loaded him up under the watchful eye of the news choppers and secured the area. Once I hooked up my headset, I heard Matt telling the other pilots where we were going and informing them we were coming up. We were going to Maricopa County Medical Center, the closest trauma center that took pediatric patients.

It didn't take us long to get there, but as we were landing we could see TV news vans already in the parking lot and set up to film us coming in. Without giving them any further attention, we got out to take our patient inside. As usual, there was a security guard and trauma nurse bringing out the stretcher to the aircraft. We slid Jeremiah on the gurney and took him into the trauma room. After giving them my report, getting my chart signed and tearing them off a copy, I headed out.

Standing just inside the door was Michael. "Would you mind talking to the press?" he asked.

I looked at him. "Whadaya mean?"

"Tell them what you did," he answered. "Let them interview you."

"I guess," I said. "There's not much to say. He had a broken arm."

"That's okay," he said. He looked over at the cameras set up out by the helipad. "They just want to get an interview. Do you mind?"

"No, I don't care. You're the PR guy. If you say it's okay, then sure, whatever."

I have never been interviewed by the press before, certainly never on camera. I am a little apprehensive. I looked at Bob.

"Do you want to do it?" I asked him.

"Hell no," he said and shied away. "I don't want all them woolies and their doohickeys staring in my face. You just go on. You can do it."

Reluctantly, I walked out to where they were all crowding around the helipad fence. Michael right beside me.

"What do I say?" I asked Michael. "What can I say? I can't give them his name."

"No," Michael agreed. "Just tell them what you picked up and what condition they were in. If they ask any questions, just answer them. But, yeah, don't give any personal information. It'll be okay, don't worry. Nothing to it."

I no sooner got up to the fence and they were already asking questions. "What happened?"

"Well," I said, trying to get some moisture into my suddenly very dry mouth, "we responded to a motor vehicle accident south of here on a dirt side road to interstate 10. The vehicle had rolled over. I don't know the reason why. We attended to a ten-year-old male who was ejected from the vehicle. He sustained a fractured arm that was stabilized on scene. We transported him here to the trauma team in stable condition."

I thought that came out pretty well, all professional without stumbling. Then the questions started.

"What happened?"

"A vehicle rolled over and the occupants were ejected."

"Do you know why the car rolled?"

"No."

"What injuries did the child have?"

"Just a fractured arm, I believe."

"What condition is he in?"

"Stable condition," I answered. I thought to myself, "Did any of you hear the report I just gave you? Was anyone actually listening, or do you all just have that 'I'm really listening to you' look pasted on your face?"

Then, without notice, not a thank you, a fuck off, or anything else, they just turned away, looked into their respective cameras and signed off. They started packing up their stuff and

I was just standing there like, "Is that it?" Michael put his hand on my shoulder and told me I did good. Then he too turned and walked away. What the hell? I thought. That came and went like a sandstorm. I turned for the helicopter and walked over.

"Well, how'd it go, superstar?" Bob said with a grin not very well hidden under his heavy moustache.

"Just get in the aircraft," I responded, not very amused.

We got back to base about 9 PM and, of course, we told everybody about the call and the news people. We had to turn on the news and watch my debut. I called my wife and told her to tape the news on different channels on both TVs we had. Matt joined us in the green room to watch it with us. Ten o'clock and sure enough, it was the lead story.

"A child critically injured tonight was flown to the trauma center following a catastrophic motor vehicle accident earlier today," reported one channel.

What! Was this the same accident I was on? Maybe they're talking about another one. Nope. They're reporting about ours.

One by one, each news channel came on giving a report about this disastrous car accident. One had the child as a three-year-old in critical condition, the other had them as a five-year-old with life threatening injuries, the other a six-year-old critically injured, the other an eight-year-old in serious condition, the closest yet, and the last had him as a four-year-old in unstable condition with multiple injuries. Then, they showed a few second clip of me, heavily edited to say a ten-year-old with a broken arm in stable condition.

You have to understand that those newscasters come into people's homes every night, giving them the real "scoop" of the day's news. Not gossip, but the facts of what happened today. These were people the general public saw every day. Someone they trusted to give them the story and details of the events happening in their city and around the world. These were trusted, honest people. Hell, most people considered newscasters damn near members of the family. They would never lie. Yet, when my clip came up with me telling them what I brought in, it made me sound like I didn't know who I had or how bad off they were, or what condition they were in. I was the one that sounded like an idiot. I was the poor shmuck they'd never seen before, why would they trust me?

I couldn't believe it. Even with the taped version of me telling them exactly what I brought into the hospital, they still got it wrong. Each and every one of them. I sat there dumbfounded.

Bob commented quietly with a gravelly voice, "That's not what I remember. Damn, must have been asleep or that was a different accident. Those do-hankies didn't even get close."

I looked around at everybody with a completely discombobulated expression. Most of my dear colleagues were quite sympathetic, as they were outright laughing at me. "Ah, don't worry that you didn't have a clue what you were doing or with who, at least you looked good."

Matt who had flown for the news channels, said, "Hey, you have to understand, they have two rules. One, don't let the facts get in the way of the story. And two, if it bleeds, it leads. If it's not newsworthy, dramatic, heart-breaking, or gory, they're not going to show it. If they're going to show it, they're going to make it newsworthy. Be thankful they showed it."

"Yeah," I said, "but I'm the one who looks like a bumbling nincompoop."

Matt shrugged, grinning.

I'm staring at the TV in utter disbelief. *Thanks a lot, Michael. Glad I could help. Call on me anytime. Happy to help out.*

I love this job. Fucking news channels.

When I got home in the morning, my wife asked me if I thought the baby was going to make it. She was serious. She was concerned about the three-year-old that she heard about. That was the one that registered with her.

I told her the truth. The real story.

"Well," she said, doubting me, "that's not what they said. You really think the kid was ten years old?"

She asked me this with complete sincerity. Like I wasn't sure of my facts. I couldn't believe it. All I could do was shake my head and go into the kitchen to make breakfast.

Chapter 10
PERSONALITIES - ABBREVIATED

I have to tell you, when you combine the medical industry and the aviation industry, you have a match made in heaven. Both of them are generally filled with class A, egotistical, over-achievers. People that strive to be the elite; the best of the best. And people who think they are the elite and the best of the best. But that's not really a bad thing. You really need people who strive for the best, that push to be above the rest, that take an immense amount of pride in being the top of the line. Otherwise, you get people who become complacent pretty quickly, and complacency in this profession will get someone killed.

Now, for those who *think* they are the best of the best, and God knows there are plenty of them that are not, they're dangerous. But, thankfully, they get weeded out reasonably fast. It's hard to hide your knowledge and skill level when you're with team members for hours even days, at a time. You sit with them, you live with them, you sleep with them. They know what you like to eat, when you go to the bathroom, how long you're in the bathroom, what your family life is like. They get to know your likes and dislikes. They get to know almost everything about you as if family members. Intimately. Personal things. Especially the medical side. We are groomed in the very personal field of healthcare. Over time, it is inevitable that we become indifferent in asking perfect strangers very personal questions that the average person would never dream of asking. How old are you? How much do you weigh? When was your last menstrual period? Are you sexually active, and if so, how much and with how many people? What drugs do you take? And, really, what drugs do you take? I'm not going to tell anyone. I'm not going to turn you in. But if you don't tell me the truth about everything, I could give you something that will kill you. Like any man having chest pain, it is imperative to know if you take Viagra and when was the last time you took it. If your shy and don't tell me because it's embarrassing, or you want to deny the need to use it. Then when I give you Nitroglycerine to relieve your chest pain, I probably just killed you. Nitro with Viagra will drop your blood pressure so far, so fast, that I will not be able to reverse the effects and you're a dead man. And then, great, I'm the one who gets in trouble for it. Thank you.

In that environment, it doesn't take long to see someone's ability and knowledge level. Now, many come in lacking that kind of skill at first. But, if you're honest, everyone will help bring you up to speed. At least most everyone. But, if you walk around thinking you're God's gift to the industry, you know everything and don't need to be told anything, then you're just begging to catch rejection. Eventually, you'll be gone. And reputation in the small circle of EMS travels quickly.

In my time, I have seen the real best of the best. I have seen nurses and medics that were far above the average, even the very good. I have also seen those that were well on their way to become the elite, with their drive and openness to learn. And, unfortunately, I have seen those who really should not even be in the medical profession at all. Let alone in a helicopter with just one other team member taking care of a critical patient.

But I have seen the best of the best everywhere. Flight crews, despite what they or anyone else thinks, are not unique, or heroes, or supreme individuals. They are medical professionals who have experience and are continually trained to do a job. A job that they worked for, wanted, applied for, and got. Ninety-nine percent of them are no more elite, however, than many I've seen on the ground, in ambulances, in hospitals, or even in clinics. They just happen to do their work in a helicopter. To be honest, there are far more people that used to work as flight crews and are now doing something else than there are current flight crews active in the field. Because of the typical personality of the medical crews you find in the field of flight, they tend to keep going on to higher degrees and working in a different environment. Helicopter transport has been around since virtually the early 1970s, the industry is still here but people age and move on or retire.

The same can be said for the pilots. They are some of the most skilled in the industry. Medical pilots don't get hired out of flight school or even with just a little experience. They're extensively trained and experienced before they can become eligible for that job. But medical flying is different than almost any other type of flying with a completely different type of crew. An egotistical crew in their own right. There is much to learn for the first-time medical pilot. New pilots are only use to talking with flight controllers and other pilots, but now they're dealing with medical issues and patients that they are unfamiliar with, flight crews that have probably flown with several experienced medical pilots prior to them and dealing with fire and police on the radio that they're not used to.

But, again, if they're up for the task, then they do great and really do become a cut above most. However, they are also scrutinized along with the rest of the team. Because, in the end, they are all one team and may, heaven forbid, die together as a team.

However, I have seen pilots that come in so full of themselves that it is a wonder how the helicopter is able to lift them and their ego off the ground. They are the pilot-in-command and everything that happens in and around and to that aircraft is their responsibility and no one else's. They are ultimately responsible for every aspect of the aircraft and the flight. No one outranks them.

Some pilots can just be impossible, though. In my full career, I have worked with over 100 of them. All but just the slightest few of them are great people, but you always have a couple in any career, including medical, who think they're above it all. Just because they are the pilot-in-command and this business is all about the helicopter, they think it's all about them.

One rule I have seen in every flight program is the "three to go, one to no" rule. Meaning, it takes all three of you, pilot, nurse and medic, to get in the aircraft and say, GO. It only takes one of you to not get in the aircraft, or to say, NO, and the mission is scrubbed. You don't even have to have a reason. You don't feel good about this mission. You don't like the weather. Something just seems off somehow. Or, the pilot, or one of the other crew members is being an ass, in some way. No questions asked. One NO and you don't go. Now, of course, someone, sometime is going to ask why. But, at the time, no questions. One NO and NO GO.

One night I had to work with a notorious pilot that others had talked about being difficult. He came in to cover the shift. I knew him but hadn't worked with him much. He was relatively new but I had been around for a while. He intimidated many of the newer medical crews with his authority. I, by this time, wasn't so easily intimidated. I had become a little saucy and jaded. I still had an immense amount of respect for what our pilots did. They were really good, and in my eyes, special. But this night I was not in the mood to endure a dictator who wanted to bully crews. I was sitting on the couch, trying to get a muscle spasm in my back to relax. Well, in comes Mr. Pilot of the Year, telling us both, the medic and me, how it's going to be this way, and how *he* expects us to perform, and what *he's* going to do and what we're not. And I had just about enough of it.

So, sitting there very quietly, I said, "I know that you're in charge of the aircraft. I respect that. I know that you're the pilot-in-command. I understand and appreciate that. I'm ready and willing to do what you ask. I'm perfectly aware that you're the big cheese, the number one, the chief, the last word, the captain and the one in charge of the aircraft." I paused for effect. "But until my *medical* butt gets in that thing, it's not an ambulance. It is just another flying fucking tour bus. And you're just another flying tour bus operator. *Comprende*?"

He stood there shocked and taken aback for a moment. I think that's when he recognized that we are all a team and each plays an equally important role to the mission and the job. It was a good night after that, partly because we ended up not getting a call during his shift. It was a little out of character for me to say that, but my back was hurting and it slipped out. But I never heard any more negative comments about him after that.

Another reason that the aviation and medical industries are a good match is that they both have a passion and a fascination for abbreviations. I don't think I've ever seen two disciplines so enthralled with abbreviating everything. Well, I take that back. When it comes to abbreviations, I don't think anyone can top the computer technology industry. But, really, they're a bunch of nerds that have been speaking a different language all of their lives and recently have forced all the normal people to educate themselves to follow suit. You seriously cannot live without them. Damn it. And especially in either the aviation or the medical industries of today. They control everything. From the aircraft instrumentation and control, to dispatching and operations, to medical charting and even drug dispensing.

The computer industry aside, aviation and medical are right up there with their love of abbreviations. Aviation with their IFR, VFR, ICS, RPM, N1, N2, so on and so forth. Medical with their MI, MVA, ICB, NC, TBI, BP, SPO2, ETCO2, again, so on and so forth. It makes them sound like their talking a completely different language and, hence, mysterious and exotic. Because most people don't understand it, that makes the aviation and medical personnel sound knowledgeable and in a different class. BS ... you know what *that* means.

It often reminds me of the line in the movie *Good Morning Vietnam* with Robin Williams, when he's talking about the impending arrival of the VIP, vice president Richard Nixon. "*Excuse me sir. Seeing as how the VP is such a VIP, shouldn't we keep the PC on the QT. Because if it leaks to the VC, he could end up an MIA and then we'd all be put on KP.*" Which, by the way, had me in tears when I first heard it and all I could think of was listening to flight crews.

Abbreviations are just the language of any profession. All

occupations have their own abbreviations and lingo. Many abbreviations in the medical profession are somewhat obvious to most people, many have been acquired through time, especially with TV shows. But some are more obscure and less often used and therefore not familiar at all. And some ... are completely made up by individual teams or groups in this business. Like most non-EMS people know that a DOA means that a person is Dead-on-Arrival. But many in the EMS field will call it a 901, which is the official designation for a death. But some of the older EMS crews talking to colleagues will say that the patient is "DRT," Dead-Right-There.

One of my favorite abbreviations is a "FDGB." Officially, dispatch would call it a "fall injury." But we would know it as a FDGB or Fall Down Go Boom. Another one we used, when we came up on a chaotic scene, where everything was a little crazy, we would call it a "Charlie Foxtrot." Which is how you say the letters C and F in aviation terms. Otherwise known to us as a "Cluster Fuck." Of course, it's not very professional to use such language, so that was just kept between the flight crews. That was our little secret. But, boy howdy, did we come up on some Charlie Foxtrots in our time!

Chapter 11
AIRFIELD CRASH

One Charlie Foxtrot that comes to mind happened up by Lake Pleasant not long after we started Native 5. There is an airfield for gliders at a place called Soaring Paradise. Their whole purpose was gliders, glider storage, glider flights, and training glider pilots. It was in a deserted area between Phoenix and Lake Pleasant out in the middle of the desert.

I was watching TV when I heard Matt say, "Scene call!"

Without a great amount of enthusiasm, Brian and I started getting ready to go. After getting rigged up in the aircraft, Matt confirmed we were ready.

"Crank the shit out of it, Matt," I said. I beat him to the punch this time.

"Shit crankin'!" he yelled back. "Make sure your trays are in the upright position, because we're getting' the hell out of Dodge." Matt was in particularly good form today. Even the takeoff had particular finesse today. Just after lifting, he tilted the aircraft hard over to the left and we flew sideways at a left angle for a moment until he brought the nose around and powered forward over the runways.

The call was for an airplane crash on the glider airport's

runway. That didn't sound good. Brian and I knew this was going to be one of those few calls that was going to put us to the test. After some time doing this job you get gut feelings about certain calls when you hear them. There is nothing in a report of an airplane crash that sounds docile. All of our knowledge and experience was going to be needed to be referenced on this one. We started getting prepped and ready right from liftoff.

Coming over the scene, we could see several fire trucks, an ambulance, and loads of people all scurrying around the patient—just one victim, not an entire plane full—a few feet away from the wreckage. Even from our height, we could see several responders around the patient with one doing CPR compressions. This was going to be bad. There was no guessing about that. It kind of looked like a little Charlie Foxtrot from where we were already.

We landed about 100 feet away so we didn't blow a bunch of debris into the scene where they were working. Quickly, as soon as we landed, we grabbed all of our stuff and headed over.

They already had the patient intubated with a breathing tube and were giving respirations with an ambu-bag. They were putting in additional IVs, doing compressions, pushing drugs and calling out everything in excited voices. The medic I was talking to was busy writing everything down interlaced with trying to give me report.

This was the pilot of one of the tow planes that takes the gliders up to altitude for launch. It was reported that the tow cable was released prematurely while still having considerable tension in the line. The cable actually snapped back and damaged the tow-plane's wing. The pilot lost control and essentially spiraled down and crashed at the wreck site. The people that were watching the event knew immediately to call 911 for assistance even before the plane hit the ground. The response was rapid. Emergency crews were on scene within minutes. Bystanders tried to extricate the pilot from the wreckage, but it took the trained firefighters to accomplish the extrication. Fearing the danger of fire, they pulled the pilot a safe distance away and started working to stabilize him.

"Clear!" I heard a rescuer shout. I looked over to see him defibrillate the patient. A brief pause to watch the monitor and then, "Continue CPR!"

You could tell, by what was being said by the obviously upset and emotional bystanders, that they knew the pilot and held him in high regard. The scene was pretty frantic. Plastic wrappers for IV bags were being thrown around. Trauma dressings flying. One rescuer desperately trying to hold the head steady while holding the intubation tube in place so it wouldn't get pulled out. While doing that, he was talking to the other rescuer who was bag breathing for the patient at a pace that was just a little rapid. Not uncommon when adrenaline is pumping off the scale.

I looked down at this poor unfortunate man lying there, thinking of what all needed to be done. As I kept looking, it was becoming clear to me that this was probably not a viable patient. The way the body was twisted led me to believe this was a lost cause. And not just the way the arms and legs were twisted, but the way the neck seemed a little skewed going from the shoulders to the head. In fact, after looking a little more closely, the torso just didn't look right either.

I asked the medic what, if anything, the patient had responded to. The medic reported that he had been completely unresponsive to anything. When they first put him on the monitor, he had an EKG tracing of about 90 beats per minute. A blood pressure of 80/50. Those readings were low but showed his heart was still beating. That really wasn't encouraging. Even after an unrevivable trauma the heart will continue to beat for some time. No respirations on their arrival, so bag and mask ventilations were started immediately. They got him secured on a backboard, got a large bore IV in and intubated right away. They have already given one and a half liters of IV fluids. Shortly after that he "coded," meaning his heart stopped and they started CPR, they gave him an amp of Epinephrine. Epinephrine is generally known to the public as adrenaline. It wasn't very long and they were able to get a heart rate back. That was just before we arrived.

"Hold CPR a minute!" the lead rescuer shouted. "Idioventricular. Give him another amp of Epi and continue CPR." The lead rescuer's voice was not completely panicked, but you could tell his own epinephrine was definitely pumping.

I noticed that even while the medic was giving compressions, the body just didn't look right. When you're pressing on the chest of a body while doing CPR, the body moves in a certain predictable response to it. Like when you push down on the chest the abdomen protrudes up. This man's chest, abdomen, hell, even his pelvic area was moving unnaturally. It was time for me to do an assessment of this patient. So, I made my way into the throng, without trying to get in the way of anybody. I straddled the patient at upper thigh and knelt down to palpate this guy's body. I might be able to feel why his body looked so wrong. As I was kneeling, I could see bloody mist coming up the intubation tube every time he was bagged. His eyes were half opened and all I could see were two big black pupils and red where white should be. That told me the impact was so severe that even his eyes were hemorrhaging.

There are somewhere around 206 bones in the human body. If this guy had two that weren't broken I'd be amazed. As I was palpating the abdomen, I could easily feel his liver was split in half. Typically, when someone is bleeding a lot into the abdomen, it becomes distended and rigid. This abdomen, on the other hand, was just mush. You could clearly feel it was full of fluid but not much left to contain it anywhere specifically. If his abdomen was in this state, I could only imagine what his heart and lungs looked like, not to mention his brain. This patient was dead.

I stood up and looked at Brian. We have worked together so long that I could read his eyes, and he could read mine. I couldn't see any reason to continue this course of action and I certainly couldn't see strapping this guy's family with an aeromedical bill for no reason. If this patient had any chance, I'd be all up in it. But sometimes you have to call a spade a spade. This man was definitely a spade.

"Hold CPR," I said. I looked at the flat line on the monitor. "You can continue CPR, but we're going to need to pronounce him."

Uh oh. Now I'd done it. I said the one thing nobody wanted to hear or do. They had put such an effort into all of this that no one wanted to give up. This team had worked feverishly to save this man's life and didn't want to be told it was all for nothing. EMS crews don't know the meaning of "give up." I knew instantly that I had just become very unpopular. And not just with the EMS crew but also with the friends of the man standing behind me. While we were doing something, that gave them some hope.

"What do you mean?" the lead medic barked. I could see about nine sets of eyes staring at me as well. Some of the stares had some fire in them.

"This guy is beyond rescue," I told him.

"But we were able to get his heart back," the rather well-built medic said, stepping a little closer to me.

"Yeah, that's the drugs. There is nothing viable here."

He didn't care for my answer or input, really. "If nothing else, he could be a donor. Don't you think?"

"No," I answered. "I don't think any of his organs would be considered for transplant."

He looked at me incredulously. Silently, standing his ground. He knew once I was on scene, I was the senior medical person, but he didn't like it.

"Look," I tried to console him, "if you palpate his abdomen, you can feel his liver is obviously split. That means that everything else is in pretty bad shape too. You guys did a very good job. I'm surprised you were able to keep him going this long. But you know in your heart, this guy is gone."

Reluctantly, he paused and looked down at the man. Then he looked around at all his coworkers staring up at him. He looked back at me with resignation in his eyes. He knew I was right.

"No chance, huh?" Now his voice was quieter and more somber. He did not want to give up, that is just not in their nature to ever give up.

"You guys did him good." I looked at him with a respectful nod. "If he had any chance, he would have had it with you guys."

Now I'm completely playing the PC card the best I can. You don't want to give these guys a bad taste for you or your team. They are still the ones that make the determination to utilize a flight company in the first place.

"Hey," I told him, "I learned a long time ago, there are just two rules to emergencies. Rule number one; people die. And rule number two; you can't change rule number one."

I got on the radio and contacted medical control and got a doctor on the line. I explained to him the situation and status and requested to pronounce the patient dead. He heartily agreed and gave me his name for the records and an official time of death.

I returned to the site. "Stop CPR." Most of the time, when I get to the point where I think it's time to pronounce, I would first ask everyone involved if they agreed. I knew in this case I probably was not going to get a unanimous response. And I didn't feel like having to discuss it or justify the decision. It was the right thing to do and I knew it.

"It was a noble try, guys. But just look at the circumstances. You did the very best. You should be proud."

I shook the big paramedic's hand and thanked him again. I could see he came around and understood. It was a tough one. I stood around for a moment to let the situation sink in and calm down, and to answer any questions that might be posed. Once it was obvious that everyone was resigned to the outcome, we gathered our equipment and headed back to the helicopter. Matt looked at us coming up without a patient. He knew what that meant. We climbed in slowly.

"Didn't make it, huh?" Matt asked, already knowing the answer.

"Nope," I responded. "That one's not a save." Even my voice was depressed.

"Good to go?" Matt asked.

"Copy."

The cockpit was quiet on the way back, humble. Matt transmitted to dispatch that we were returning to base. He then talked to air traffic control for return to base. Once we were back on the ground at base, he asked more about the case and what happened. Most of the pilots are curious and interested in what medical does and why. Matt was particularly interested, but in this case, he was also respectfully brief. Matt was just good people. Yeah, you don't come across anybody better than Mrs. Uhl's little boy.

Chapter 12
SHIT HAPPENS

In this business, there are times when your whole shift is a shut-out. You won't get a call for the entire twenty-four hours. That can make for a long day. It's more common in the summer months than the winter. Part of that has to do with less people living in the heat of Arizona. Phoenix has a high "snow-bird" population. People who just live there in the winter to get out of the snow from back home, wherever that may be. Some of it is due to the fact that less people get out and mill around in the extreme heat. They just stay inside with the air-conditioning. But that's not necessarily a bad thing, because that just means we don't have to get out in the heat either.

Just sitting on the tarmac all day, the helicopter gets pretty hot inside. We generally have an external air-conditioner hooked up, blowing cold air into the cabin which helps tremendously. But, as soon as you disconnect it, the cabin starts to heat up rapidly. It doesn't take long for it to be back over a hundred degrees in there. Helicopter air-conditioning systems are notorious for not doing a very good job. There's a whole lot of window area, much like a green-house, which is necessary to have good visualization, but it's not very conducive for cooling.

Plus, the ports for the air-conditioning are small and sparse.

So, we are not too upset when we don't have to get out in the heat of the day to run calls. IFTs, or interfacility transfers, are not as bad because you are picking up a patient in a cool hospital environment and taking them over to another cool hospital environment. Not so bad, except the helicopter is shut down while you're in the facility packing and unpacking the patient. The longer the helicopter is not running and just sitting there, the hotter it gets. Scene calls, on the other hand, you're working out in the elements and sweating your ass off, but the helicopter is kept running thus keeping the interior as cool as it can. There are pros and cons to everything.

Most people think that you do a lot of scene calls during rush hour traffic. But the truth is quite opposite. The fact is, during rush hour traffic, that in reality is about four hours in the morning and about four hours in the evening, we don't get called much. Not for MVAs anyway. During rush hour, a lot of cars are getting into accidents, that's true. But, there are so many of them crammed on the road that they can't really get going very fast. So, what you end up with is a whole lot of bent metal and not many injuries. No, we get the calls after and in-between rush hour when everybody is still in the "hurry up" mode and there is far fewer vehicles thus creating much larger spaces when they can get going much faster. Some people just have the uncontrollable need to zip in and through those open spots, like it's actually going to do some good and save time. It really doesn't. Very few people driving today are trained at high-speed maneuvering, even though everyone thinks they are. When they finally find out they are not good at it is when they smack something really hard and do a great deal of damage. That's when we get the calls.

When Brian and I came in, we got the report from the off-going team that they were shut out during their shift. The team the day before had the same shut out. Bummer for us, kind of, because that just increased our chances that we were going to get some calls. It's just the odds. Shut outs can't go on forever, but we could hope.

We went through the morning with our same routine. Counting the narcotics first, so the off-going crew could go home. Brian and I checked equipment, did the necessary paperwork, went out to the aircraft before the morning heat set in and checked it out. Mike was already out there doing his routine pre-flight check of the aircraft. When we got back inside and all the business duties were taken care of, we went about our own personal routines. I zapped a breakfast biscuit in the microwave and went in to lay down and watch some TV.

Usually, if we were going to get a call, it would be around 10 AM to about 1 PM. The chances may go up around 3 PM for an IFT. The time we were more likely to get a call was after 8 PM to about 2 or 3 AM. For our base, that just seemed to be about normal. But everything in this business is about the unexpected. You just never know when you're going to get a call or what it might be for. Nothing in EMS is predictable. So, if you're smart, you stay prepared. For me, that meant taking a nap in the morning when I knew our chances of being called were at the lowest, typically. That way I'd be ready for any 3 AM calls.

This day was normal. About 3 PM we received a dispatch for a call out of Maryvale Hospital for a cardiac patient. Maryvale was in one of the seedier parts of town. Generally, the calls we get are either cardiac related for the older people, or very often trauma related to gang violence in the proximity. Gunshot wounds, were not uncommon, along with stabbings and beatings.

This turned out to be a heart attack. The guy was fifty-eight years old and started having chest pain that morning but he just thought it was indigestion. By 2 PM he decided to have it checked out. If a man is finally deciding to have his "indigestion" checked out at a hospital, he is either really hurting or is really scared or both. So, he came in and, sure enough, he was having a heart attack, which is caused by blood clotting in some narrowed coronary arteries, the main blood vessels of the heart. They gave him aspirin to prevent the blood from clotting further. That's what aspirin does.

Years ago, when I was a new nurse, the first time I had a doctor tell me to give a heart attack patient aspirin, I thought, "Jeez, dude. It's a heart attack! I think I'd give him a little more than a couple of aspirin and have him call me in the morning."

As for our man at Maryvale Hospital, after the aspirin they started him on a Nitroglycerine IV drip. As opposed to just giving Nitro under the tongue. It can be controlled much better that way. The Nitro helps relieve the pain by relaxing the blood vessels to the heart. Which is why the heart is screaming with pain, it's starving for blood and oxygen. But Nitro can also lower the blood pressure significantly, so giving it via IV is a much better way to control pain without dropping the blood pressure too much. They also gave him some Morphine to just really kick start some pain relief.

By the time we got there, the man was pain-free and doing good. They just wanted him transferred to "Good Sam" hospital for cardiac care and a cardiac catherization lab. No biggy for us, we just loaded him up and zipped him over there. The hardest part about this call was the charting. I love taking care of patients but charting everything you did, everything the hospital did, everything the patient did or said, everything that should be done, everything everybody thinks, every bird you pass en route, this, that, and everything else, what a pain. I hated charting. Every chart you write was critiqued by no less than three people after the call. And, it seemed, everybody's got to give you their input. *Well, did you think of this? Well, did you do that? If not, why? You did this, why?* I hated quality assurance. It demanded that every chart be scrutinized for proper care of the patients and job quality. While, I know it was necessary, that didn't mean I had to like it. It was still a pain in the ass. In all honesty, the hardest part of ninety-nine percent of our calls was the charting, not the care or the pressures. In truth, I felt more pressure from charting than patient care. By this time, for the most part, taking care of patients was instinctive. It was the fun part of the job, the challenge. But, then again, if everything about the job was fun, the company would probably try to get you to pay them to do it.

The sun was still blazing above the horizon when we got back to base. I went in to finish the paperwork while Brian straightened up and restocked the aircraft and Mike refueled. As soon as they came in the doors, the Nextel went off. We got a call out of Boswell Hospital in Sun City for a pediatric patient with respiratory distress. What the hell was a pediatric patient doing in a retirement community hospital? Boswell Hospital was in a massive retirement community but it served the entire area. It is a great hospital so, everybody went there. But they didn't have a definitive pediatric unit. So, call in NAAA to transport the child to Phoenix Children's Hospital, where they belong.

A pediatric patient in respiratory distress. This could be interesting. How little is the kid? How serious is the condition? This could test your knowledge and abilities. Children can often be very challenging because of their nature and the fact they can mask just how severe the problem is until the very end. Kids have incredible reserve capabilities. They can be pretty sick for a long time but look perfectly normal until, suddenly, they just give out. Then all hell breaks loose, because by that time you are so far behind the eight-ball you have a hell of a time catching up. If you can at all. You have to be alert with kids and always be ahead of them. You have to really look at them closely, how they're reacting to all the commotion going on around them. If they're screaming and crying, that's a good sign. If they're quiet and uninterested, letting everybody do what they need to do, like start IVs, without much fuss, then you have a very critical child. I don't care what the monitor might be reading. Yeah, this could be interesting.

We got to Boswell Hospital and went in to get report. This was a male, eight years old with a history of asthma. He came in with respiratory distress. He was wheezing with sternal retractions and had a hard time catching his breath. They had given him a couple of breathing treatments that helped remarkably well and now he was no longer wheezing or panting. But they still wanted him transferred to Phoenix Children's Hospital for further evaluation and care. Routine. He's getting the breathing treatments on a continuous basis, and they wanted him monitored by a nurse. That's where we come in. He's not really what you would call critical, but that's what the hospital wanted. You call, we haul. I'm not going to question it. Mine is not to reason why, mine is just to do the job. Besides, he could still always turn bad again quickly.

We packaged the boy on our gurney, hooked him up to the monitors, put his breathing treatment on our oxygen tank, and headed out. Not much to it. Again, it's all about the chart. This guy really could have gone by ground ambulance. Completely uneventful.

We dropped him off and headed back to base. Mike was running out of time that he could still fly, according to FAA regulations. He was on a twelve-hour shift and can fly up to fourteen hours, but then he turns into a pumpkin and can no longer fly. FAA rules. He was within the window right now so he had enough time to return to base without a problem. As soon as we got back he reported off with Bud.

I finished the paperwork, hoping that was the last call for the shift, and faxed the chart to the main office. That gets the billing ball rolling. It's imperative that the paperwork get to the billing office as soon as possible for them to do their job and get reimbursement for the flight. This may be a "caring" business, but it was still a business. Payment had to be received or the whole thing just stopped. That's business.

Bud came in after finishing his pre-mission stuff and the three of us chatted for a bit. We've all been working together for a few years, since we started the base. Brian, Bud, and I have been here since the beginning. In fact, almost everyone at this base has been here since the beginning. Native 5 was affectionately known as the "vacation station" because of the other aeromedical company below us generally took half the calls out of this area. It was a contractual arrangement the companies had with Phoenix Alarm, the emergency dispatching center. We were on an "every other call" schedule with the other company for emergency scene calls. Hospitals could still call whoever they wanted. The effect was that we generally didn't have as many monthly calls as some other bases. We were also known as the "retirement" base, because all the flight crews here were here from the start and we didn't leave until we were going to retire. Hell, Bud was at retirement age and was still hanging on. Many people wanted to work Native 5 but until someone retired, or died, there just wasn't an opening. So, tough luck.

Brian and I had already changed into our more comfortable evening attire and were getting ready to relax. Brian and Bud were sitting in the living area chatting, with me in the kitchen area putting a TV dinner in the microwave. The living area and the kitchen area are only separated by the counter that the computer, phone, fax machine, and other business essentials were on. One side was kept clear to be used for a place to eat. Otherwise, it was essentially just a big combined room. Brian was just about to turn on the TV and my dinner had about two more minutes to cook when the Nextel came alive. I didn't pay much attention to it this time because it was about the time dispatch would routinely check in for evening roll call. But, not this time, it was to dispatch us on a mission. Shit. My dinner was only half cooked.

"Really!" I said in feigned exasperation. You can act like it's an inconvenience, but it really is just the job.

It was for an MVA up on Interstate 17, just north of Black Canyon City. Roll-over MVA with extrication in progress.

"An extrication, huh?" I said as I cancelled the microwave. We got ready and hurried to the aircraft. More often than not, when someone had to be extricated, they generally had significant traumatic injuries. We got in the aircraft and got secured.

"All set?" Bud asked.

"Yup, good to go," I replied. Not wasting any time, Bud was off.

It was about 8:30 PM and the small airport wasn't busy at this time. During the day, it could sometimes take a few minutes to get clearance to lift. Deer Valley Airport was a busy airport during the day for various reasons. Sometimes, it could take some time to even get a radio break to contact the tower for permission to lift. Luckily, not tonight at this time.

Bud received clearance immediately to cross the runways and head north. Shortly after getting underway, we received word that the victim in the MVA was pregnant. She was the one they were trying to extricate. That wasn't good. When Brian and I first got in the aircraft, with the way the day had been already, we thought this was going to be another "bone call." That's what we referred to a call that was just a routine, run-of-the-mill, nothing to be done, "why did you call for an aircraft?" type of call. Flight personnel are the type that want the go-get- em, test-your-wits, blood and guts, gritty, down and dirty, be-a-hero kind of calls. When you don't get that, which happened a lot, you feel kind of like you got boned. This didn't sound like it was going to be a bone call.

"We have about twenty-six minutes in flight," Bud informed us.

"Shit," I uttered. "This time, that could be important."

"I'm peddling as fast as I can," Bud came back over the intercom. "I'm not as young as I used to be, you know." Bud was not in any way apologetic about his age. He was older and proud of it. The crews like to make fun of it, though, but all in jest. And Bud was a great sport.

"I appreciate that, Bud." I waited for just a second, then added, "Just don't have a frickin' heart attack on us. I mean, if you even start to look bad, I'm not going to check you out, use IV drugs, or even start CPR. I'm going straight to electricity. I'm gonna shock the shit out of ya."

"Yeah," Brian popped in. "I'm not doing mouth to mouth on you, either. I like you and all, but there's lines I won't cross."

"Hey, and I brushed my teeth just for you too. You know, I …" Bud was interrupted by the radio clicking on.

"Native 5, what's your ETA to the scene?" dispatch queried. "Fire is requesting."

It's pretty unusual for fire to request an ETA while you were en route unless you were well overdue. When a flight request was originally made, our dispatcher would give them the estimated time for us to arrive on scene. If they were wanting to know while we were still well within that time frame, it generally meant they were getting inpatient. That's never a good sign. I gave Brian a look, and he gave it right back at me.

"I'm showing eighteen minutes to go," Bud responded.

"Copy that."

"Do we have any further patient information?" I asked dispatch over the radio.

"Pregnant female involved in a roll-over MVA being extricated at present. Nothing further at this time," dispatch replied.

"Copy." I ended the call. I'd like to know more. I wanted to know what I was walking into. Typically, though, you deal with what you have when you get it.

Usually, you can see the scene of an MVA from quite a few miles out by all the flickering lights after the sun goes down. Not in this case. The accident happened just as the interstate started to come down the pass through the hills after Sunset

Point rest area. We probably wouldn't be able to see the scene until we were almost right over it. After a while, I started to see a line of headlights highlighting the interstate snaking back up towards the rest area and flashes of red and blue in the air. We came around one of the peaks on the other side of the hill and there it was.

The scene was massive. Fire trucks before and after the scene on the road, at least three police cars at the scene, one south of the scene, and an ambulance right in the middle. There were two Department of Public Safety vehicles north of the scene blocking the two-lane interstate, and that's where the line of car headlights started. That line of white lights extended back at least five miles, without exaggeration. Where we were on the interstate, there was no other way around this. Interstate 17 is the only main road into Phoenix from the north. When it gets blocked for any amount of time, the back-up can extend for many miles.

From our vantage point, it was really easy to take in the whole scene. The vehicle they were working on was upside-down in the middle of the interstate. It looked like at one time it was probably an SUV, but now it appeared to be a stepped-on aluminum can. Apparently, it lost control coming around one of the bends, and with the choice of trying to climb a sheer rock face or launching over a several hundred-foot drop off, she had taken the climb the sheer rock face option. Without knowing what kind of an SUV, or if it even was an SUV, I suspected it didn't have what it needed to climb the wall. It went up so far and rolled over. More precisely, it pancaked on its roof in the middle of the road.

Bud did a couple of orbits checking out the landing zone they wanted us in, just south of the last fire truck between that and the DPS car farther down. It was kind of a tricky spot on the road with the rock face right there but very doable for Bud. It wasn't the best you could hope for, but it was the best you were going to get. After a couple of orbits Bud started to bring it in. While he was doing his orbits, I watched the scene and noticed that they were no longer in the process of extrication. They must already have the patient out and treating her somewhere. I suspected the ambulance.

Bud put Little Girl on the road without a problem. Brian and I grabbed our stuff and headed over. We were directed to the ambulance, where I already suspected the patient was being treated.

There were three medics inside caring for the patient. They must have just gotten her in the ambulance when we arrived. She was on a backboard but that was about it, they just started working on her. One of the medics was giving me report while everyone else was aiding the patient who was moaning in pain. One was cutting her clothes off, one was hooking her up to the monitor, the other was helping Brian assess the damage. I looked down at the girl who was very pregnant.

"What's your name?" I asked her. Trying to focus her on something other than all the chaos going on around her.

"Shanika," she answered. You could see her trying to maintain some control. This woman was a trooper. Most people would just be freaking out and screaming bloody murder. To hell with trying to keep composed.

"How far along are you?" I asked, trying to keep eye contact with her through the space between the legs of the medics.

She looked at me in obvious pain. "About thirty-six weeks," she gasped out.

"Do you have any children already? If so, how many?"

"I have three other children."

Shit! That means she was no stranger to giving birth. The more children you have, generally, the easier it is to deliver. This event could very easily cause premature labor. Well, that was one thing to try to prevent. Thankfully, she was answering my questions quickly and accurately despite the distress she was in. That was a good sign.

I looked at the patient while getting the report, occasionally writing some information on my tape. Two of the medics were finishing cutting her clothes off so we could get good exposure of the injuries. The left arm was obviously fractured judging by the unusual angular bend in the mid-upper arm and possibly dislocated at the shoulder. It, too, looked out of sorts. There was no mistaking the mid shaft fracture of the right thigh. Not with that bone sticking out of the skin. It was a wonder that this woman wasn't screaming uncontrollably.

Brian told me he was going to put a sager splint on the right leg. A sager splint is a traction device that attaches to the hip area and around the ankle. Once attached, you can extend it and stretch the leg down and take the tension out of the big thigh muscles that are pulling the leg together where the bone is broken and causing pain. The sager traction splint, when in place, provides much better pain control than any amount of medication I could give her. At the same time, the other medic was splinting the left arm. They already had her on the monitor and I could see, by the heartrate and blood pressure, that she was in significant pain, but other than that, she was doing good. Her heart rate was up but where I would expect it to be, and the blood pressure was holding at an acceptable reading. Oxygen saturation was doing really good too. While she was exposed right then, I briefly looked down at her vaginal area to see if there was any obvious bleeding that could indicate a traumatic problem with the pregnancy. Thankfully, nothing.

Just about the time Brian was ready to pull traction on the sager splint, I grabbed the doppler that we brought with us this time. Normally, the doppler, a little ultrasound device used to hear the baby's heartbeat, was left in the helicopter. But, knowing we had a pregnant patient we thought to bring it along. Fetal heart tones are important to note in order to have an idea how the baby is responding to all this excitement. Once in the helicopter, even with the doppler, fetal heart tones would be all but impossible to acquire.

As I was squirting gel on the end of the doppler, Brian started pulling traction and I watched the bone that was sticking up through the thigh submerge back under the skin. Just as soon as it looked straight, Shanika instantly eased up. Still in considerable pain but now much more tolerable. While I was listening to her enormous belly, one of the paramedics was bandaging the open wound on the thigh that the protruding bone had made.

I had to move the doppler around a bit to find the right spot to hear the baby's heartbeat. As I was looking, I noticed a pretty significant red mark across her lower abdomen that could have only been made by the seatbelt that jerked on her as she launched in her seat. That's not good. There is someone right below that abdomen there slamming into that belt also, the baby. Sliding the doppler around, I started to hear what I was looking for. Found it. *Clip, clop, clip clop, clip, clop*, yup, just what I wanted to hear. I counted the beats to make sure I was hearing the baby and not the mother. Mother's heartrate was 128 and the baby was clicking away at about 156. Just what I would expect. That was a relief, baby seemed to be none for the worse, so far.

While all this was going on, another medic was opening and priming an IV bag and getting the start kit out to get a very necessary IV put in. Two large bore IVs needed to be put in her since she was going to need fluids. She had not one but two broken bones. You can lose a lot of blood from broken bones. Even if the blood doesn't come out, it can be lost inside the body tissue and cause an immense drop in blood pressure, which is the last thing you want with anyone. Especially, someone who's trying to feed two bodies with the same blood supply. Plus, it was the only avenue to give her drugs.

I prepared equipment to put in the second IV. As I looked down trying to determine where to put in another IV, I realized it's not ideal to put an IV in an arm that is broken unless you can go above the break. In this case, the break was pretty high up the arm, not to mention a possible dislocation. That meant the right arm was going to be the lucky recipient of at least a couple of needle jabs. And wouldn't you know it, the right arm was up against the wall on the other side of the ambulance from where we were. Shit! That meant that getting into position to start an IV was going to be an exercise in acrobatic agility. Thankfully, women in this stage of pregnancy generally have engorged veins and are reasonably easy to stick. Graciously, she had very nice veins, and two pretty large bore IV needles were stuck in pretty quickly. That was easy. Thank the universe and mother Earth. We had one thing going for us, finally.

She was still in a substantial amount of pain, so pain medicine was definitely on the menu. Knowing what you can give someone, who was giving some of that to a baby was part of the job.

"Are you allergic to anything," I asked her.

"Penicillin," she reported. "That's all."

Well, I was not going to start her on antibiotic therapy out here right now. I pulled out my drug box and started drawing up some pain medication and an anti-nausea drug to give her. Traumatized patients are already prone to get nauseated, especially pregnant patients, but when you put a narcotic on top of that and then move them all around, not to mention fly them into the air, ... well, you get the point. Go on and give them something to help keep them from getting sick. Not only is it better for them, vomiting has very bad consequences, especially when you're strapped down to a board and can't get up, but it's also better for us. I didn't want to deal with a vomiting patient and Brian didn't want to clean it up. Neither did I.

"I'm going to give you something for the pain right now," I told her, smiling. Giving her that "everything is going to be okay" look. Out of prudence, I gave the antiemetic first, waited a second or two, then followed it with the narcotic.

Last thing to do was get her transferred over to our monitor and go. Brian was already at it and almost finished. Okay, we'd been there long enough.

Everybody got ready and we were out the door to the aircraft. I went on ahead to get everything ready. We started to load her into the aircraft, and being pregnant, that meant it was unadvisable to lay her flat. With her uterus full of baby, laying flat tends to impede blood flow back to the heart from all that weight pushing down on the main vessel returning blood to the heart. It's recommended, not to mention it was our protocol, to lean the patient on her left side to take the pressure off the vena cava, that large vessel returning blood. But that was the side she had a broken arm and possibly a dislocation. Plus, the way the aircraft was set up, that put her leaning away from us, making it harder to see her and tend to her if she did get sick. Well, it is what it is. We rolled up a couple of towels and put them under the backboard to lean her over to her left side. I'd really like to know what the baby's fetal heart tones were right now, but that was impossible with the helicopter. All I would hear with the doppler right now would be something akin to a chainsaw running. I just had to go off what I could ascertain by looking at her and watching her vital signs on the monitor. And, above all, get her to the trauma unit as quick as possible. I didn't want her in this helicopter one second longer than she needed to be.

While Brian was getting in, I got close to her face so she could hear me.

"You're going to be just fine," I hollered over the noise. "Did that pain medicine help any?"

She nodded.

"Good. If you feel like you need more, raise your right arm up and we'll try to get you fixed up." I patted her right shoulder gently and gave her a reassuring nod. "I'm going to close the door now, but I'll be right behind you."

I closed and secured the door and went around to the right side. As soon as we were ready, Bud lifted Little Girl up into the air and headed straight for John C. Lincoln Medical Center.

The flight was essentially uneventful. Shanika raised her hand one time to let us know the pain was getting worse. Without hesitation, I gave her another reasonable dose of Fentanyl. The problem with bone fractures is that it's almost impossible to get a patient pain free with medication alone. They really need to have the bone set and stabilized to get real relief. But medication should, at least, help.

Concerned about the welfare of the baby, I finally leaned

over to Shanika's ear and said loudly, "I'm going to put my hand on your belly. I want to see if I can feel the baby move, okay?"

She nodded understanding and approval.

I laid my hand on her belly for a moment, wondering just what the chances really were of me being able to distinguish fetal movement from helicopter vibration. Then, all of the sudden, I felt a push. That was an undeniable foot pushing back on my hand. Alright, that made me happy. Little punkin was pissed off. I love it. And doesn't seem to be too doped up either. Right on.

Just as we were about five minutes out, I noticed that her blood pressure was steadily falling. Not too dramatic, but definitely noticeable. I looked at her right thigh and realized it had grown considerably in size. She was bleeding into her thigh. Over and above the problems of blood loss into the tissue with hypotension, you also run into problems with circulation beyond the point of swelling to the lower leg and foot. The situation didn't have any good scenarios. She needed to get to trauma, now. Then I noticed a couple of abnormal heartbeats on the EKG monitor. Not many, but enough to get my attention. All I needed was for her to have circulatory blood problems. When the pregnant body starts to have problems, it sacrifices the fetus first. So, if Mom starts to have noticeable problems, then the baby is probably already being compromised.

I calmly put her IV bag in a pressure device and pumped it up to force IV fluids in a little faster. Brian was doing the same thing to the other bag. Fluids and more fluids.

We were coming over John C. Lincoln Hospital, I looked down at the helipad and saw another helicopter just starting to spin up with the crew getting onboard. Even though there were a couple of helipads for this hospital, it's bad form to land when another helicopter is just starting up and getting ready to take off. We'd just have to orbit for a minute, make contact with the other pilot and allow them to clear.

That would delay our off-loading. "Darn!" I just stared down there resigned. It was what it was.

"Shit," Brian mumbled.

Oh, yeah, that's it. Shit!

The other helicopter finally took off after what seemed like forever. We landed and swiftly moved to get Shanika unloaded and into trauma. I ripped out report over the din of everyone there. On this patient, there were two teams standing by ready to go; the trauma team and a neonatal/OB team. Common procedure for this type of patient. Just in case.

Everything moved pretty quick. At one point, try as I may, I could not see Shanika at all for all the bodies hovering over her. I had the receiving nurse sign my report and I stepped out of the way. Let that tornado of people do their job and we would get our equipment, monitor, and sager splint back in a bit. Brian and I dashed into the EMS room to down a quick bottle of water and returned. Just in that time, she had already gone to CT for a scan of her fractures. The only thing left in the room was a war zone of debris laying around on the floor, our monitor and sager splint off to the side. Brian wiped them down and packed them up while I went to the desk to give them a copy of my report and get a copy of their face sheet, or information sheet, for our records.

Shanika turned out to be one of those time-sensitive responses. Had she been transported in to this trauma unit by ground, it would have taken too long with the way she was bleeding. She would have lost blood pressure and needed more drastic measures to keep her going. Forget the fact that she would have been bouncing all the way to the hospital, the road vibrating and jostling her fractures. Not to mention, the effect it would have had on the baby. It could have been devastating. Yeah, this was a legitimate flight needing that intervention within the golden hour.

"Well," I exhaled, "that's a save."

We took a few more steps and I noticed Brian stop suddenly. Did he happen to catch sight of another attractive female somewhere in the emergency department? I looked at him and he was just staring at me.

"What?"

"Is that a save?" he said. "Or is that two saves?" After a moment of contemplation. "Or, would that be considered one and a half saves?"

I peered at him in consideration. *Hmm*, I thought. *That's a good question.*

"I'm calling it two," Brian stated, nodding. "Hell yeah, that's definitely two saves."

"I'll take that," I responded. "I'd think we could safely say a twofer without being too presumptuous."

We were feeling pretty good about ourselves right now, but we knew we didn't do anything special. Same thing anyone else in our shoes would've done. We had the equipment, we had the know-how, and best of all, we had the helicopter. But, we were going to bask in the momentary glory anyway.

"That's right, we bad," Brian exclaimed, starting to strut.

Gettin' down with my bad self, I followed that with, "Shiiiit!"

Chapter 13
PR

During the early years of NAAA, we did a lot of public relations events. We were trying to get our name out there and let people see who we were and what we offered. These PR events were anything from an opening of a new store to a children's toy drive to a neighborhood health and welfare event. We'd bring in the helicopter and stand around for a few hours, showing off the aircraft and answering questions. Occasionally, we'd let the little kids with their sticky, cotton-candy fingers crawl through the helicopter and see what it was like. Parents loved to get pictures of their kids in a helicopter. I don't know that Little Girl much cared for it, but she would sit there like a good little helicopter and take it. She knew we would clean her up.

You'd be surprised, however, how many little tykes would absolutely go hysterical when they got close to the bird. I don't mean happy either. They'd be crying and screaming, trying to crawl out of Mommy or Daddy's arms to get away. The thing just frightened the hell out of some of them for reasons that are still beyond my comprehension. I found it a little humorous, actually. Not because I'm unsympathetic or evil, but while they all loved helicopters flying through the air, up close it frightened them. Even kids to whom Mommy and Daddy would say, "They just love helicopters," would squirm away from their arms when they got close. It was crazy.

The first few years of PR events I went to were pretty fun. There I am, Mr. Flight Nurse, in my really cool flightsuit, looking all professional and ready to answer any questions. But like anything else, after several years it got boring. Here I am, Mr. Fucking Flight Nurse, in my cool flightsuit. Yeah, I'm a professional, what do you want to know?

Don't get me wrong, it was still fun. Once you arrived at the event, the wonder of the job washed over you with the enthusiasm of the people coming up to see what you did and asking questions. Albeit, it was the same questions over and over. All the organizers of the events were really nice too. Giving us free food and drinks, very appreciative of us coming out, and catering to our every need. Some events were really fun. Like we had the contract for a few years to be the helicopter on standby at the Phoenix International Raceway. That was a blast, especially for NASCAR week but I'm a race fan, so that helped. We sat on the field the whole time the race was underway. We could walk around anywhere because we had radios to alert us if we were needed. The pit lane, the grand stands, the garages, everywhere. Our flightsuits were worth about $1,200 dollars. The price of a VIP ticket to allow the same access, but we could do even more. Plus, we flew in and parked in the middle of the field. How cool was that? This job had its perks. But on the flip side, it also had its downsides. It was really fun to be noticed and recognized everywhere you went, but at the same time, it was also a burden to be noticed and recognized everywhere you went. If you wanted to smoke a cigarette, you were going to have at least fifty people watching you, and some of them children. So, you didn't. If you tripped on something, people noticed.

Then there were the questions. You had to interact with the public. Being medical professionals, the general public is naturally relaxed around you and feel very at ease. For some reason, we are very approachable. Some people may feel a little uneasy just walking up to a cop standing there and starting a conversation. But it seems nobody feels uneasy walking up to a firefighter or medical person and just starting up a conversation. Many times, it started out with, "You know, last year I had to call the ambulance because I fell off the roof. You guys were great," or, "Three years ago my uncle Tom was flown by helicopter after a car wreck. Maybe it was you guys. Do you remember something like that?" I always wanted to say something like, "Uh, yeah, I remember him. Kind of an older guy with short brown hair." Just to see what kind of reaction I would get. Like, "Hell yeah, that's him. So, it *was* you guys!"

But my partner would never let me do that. If it was Bob or Brian, they'd say, "You'll just get them started. They'll answer with, 'No, he was a short guy with gray hair. You got to remember him. He said you guys were the greatest.' And they'll just keep on going. Don't get them started. Please!" Sometimes, my partners were real kill-joys. I was just playing, jeez.

When we would go to these PR events, we would generally just stand by the helicopter to show the aircraft and our equipment and field questions anybody would have about our job. The most common question most people would ask is, "What's the hardest thing about your job?"

My standard answer would be, "Trying to figure out what channel I want to watch on TV." Which, in essence, would be the hardest thing I had to do. Trying to figure out how to stay entertained over the many tedious hours of waiting for a call.

Routinely, the hardest part of the job was charting accurately and quickly. On the day-to-day basis, that was the hardest part. But in reality, I couldn't really explain the hardest part of the job. Because, in truth, the hardest part of the job was listening to the wails and laments of family when you were trying to revive their loved one or feeling the need to stop resuscitation and pronounce a patient dead when you knew your attempts were futile or looking in the eyes of a parent and telling them you were not able to save their child. That was without question the hardest part of the job. But how do you explain that to someone who has never had to do something like that? It's unexplainable and incomprehensible. So, I just always replied with, "Trying to figure out what channel I want to watch." That was just easier.

Invariably, the next question asked was, "What's the worst thing you ever saw?" That's almost impossible to answer. What do you mean by the "worst thing?" The most gruesome? The most horrible, the bloodiest, the most heartbreaking? What do you mean? In any case, it's not something I really want to talk about. In most cases, it's not something that I *could* talk about. Generally, it's something that I would really not want to remember even if I could talk about it. I cannot adequately explain the worst thing I ever saw nor would I want to. In my career, I've treated and transported over 2,500 patients. How am I to pick out the worst one?

That was not specific to me, either. I guarantee you, every single person that's been in the medical profession for two years or longer has at least one "war story" of the most intriguing, gruesome, horrifying, disturbing, or heartbreaking in nature. A minimum of one. Every single medical professional. From EMT to MD. It's just the nature of the business.

To be honest with you, police, firefighters, and paramedics have the best stories. They get there first. When it's really awful, gruesome, or horrible, it's generally fatal and we, the flight crews, don't get called in. They are the ones that see the very worst of the worst. They tromp through the unmentionable to get to the very heart of the scene. Most of the time the flight crew were the second or third ones on the scene. The scene had already been made safe. Sanitized. The patient had already been identified and was, generally, already being treated. Flight crews don't generally see the really gruesome, bloody, horrific, disturbing sights. Generally.

But on occasion ...

Chapter 14
DON'T LOSE FACE

It was about two o'clock in the morning. You know, when all the bars close. This was back in my early years when I was still working at Native 1. My partner was Mike Q. Another Mike in the company. A short, dark-haired Italian guy who I loved so much, I just wanted to put him in my pocket and take him home with me. I made a stupid comment one day about how Hitler was really good for Germany in the very early years, when they were struggling after World War I, before he got too much power and became crazy. Well then, he let me have it! "You do know I'm Jewish, right?" Oops. I felt like shit, but he knew it was just the way I was, I couldn't help it, and he was the forgiving sort. Gratefully, he didn't hold it against me. He was the consummate professional paramedic. Knowledgeable, skilled, unpretentious, and efficient. He also handled all the supplies for the entire company. He knew what everything was, what it was for, and where to get it.

In those days, each person on the rotor crew carried a hand-held radio. All of the sudden two radios toned out. "Native 1 scramble. Native 1 scramble." We jogged out to the aircraft. Little Girl was sitting there patiently waiting on her crew. Matt Uhl was the pilot and was ready.

"Native 1 scramble. Native 1 scramble," the radio called out again. "Gilbert and Thomas road for a GSW." That told us about where we were going and what for. GSW, or gun-shot wound. This should be good. Good for us is not good for the patient. That was back when we were all hyped up about saving lives and eager to get down and dirty. Hell yeah, gun-shot wound. This was real emergency medical service. We were pumped. Gunshot wounds, major traumas, and the like is what emergency medical people live for, it challenges us. It put us to the test of what we've been trained and practiced for. It may be morbid, but it's what we want to do. It's when we feel like we really make a difference.

Mike and I jumped in and secured ourselves. Matt, cool as ever, methodically got in and started his routine. After checking with us and our status I heard, "Cranking the shit out of it." Mike and I had big shit-eating grins on our faces. In the tradition of the Blues Brothers, it's the middle of the night, we have a full tank of gas, we're going to a GSW and we're all wearing headsets. "Let's hit it!"

It was easy to see the scene from quite a distance out. Not unexpectantly, there were more than the usual amount of blinding red and blue lights flashing. This was a GSW, so in addition to the usual fire trucks and ambulances, there were a lot of police cars all lining the streets.

Matt made contact with the ground crew, got landing instructions and was informed that the scene was safe, an important tidbit of information when there are firearms involved. The landing zone they had laid out for us was well defined. Matt made one quick observation orbit and brought her in to land. Already prepared, Mike and I popped out and headed to the scene, where we found about twenty people standing. The police were keeping the neighbors at a distance, away from the scene. It seemed all the commotion had the whole neighborhood out and gawking.

The unfortunate victim of an apparent suicide, the man was lying facing down in the front yard of his house by a tree. The scene stuns me for a second. The man was not actually face down in the lawn. He was on his belly, resting on his elbows with his head up. There were about six firefighters and paramedics standing and kneeling around him, just staring. What in the hell was going on here? Mike went over to the victim and I made my way to the guy with the clipboard.

"What's up?" I asked.

"Well," he started off. "This is Oscar Hernandez. He's a thirty-eight-year-old male. About hundred-and-eighty pounds. Attempted suicide with a shotgun." He turned to look at me, "The neighbors heard the shotgun blast about twenty minutes ago, came out and saw him, then called 911."

I looked over and saw Mike talking to the patient and the guy's head nodding.

"When we got here," the medic continued, "we found the guy lying, pretty much where he is now. He's alert and oriented. Well, the best we can tell. He's answering appropriately, anyway. And he's essentially stable."

From my vantage point, all I could see was a guy lying on his belly, looking up at Mike and nodding. What's the catch?

"Where's the gun-shot wound to?" I asked the medic.

"To the face," he said, without batting an eye.

What? Wait a minute. To the face? And everyone's just standing around?

"To the face?" I reiterated. There's no hiding the questioning surprise in my voice. "And, he's alert?" I was still unable to conceal my astonishment. "What are his vital signs?" I asked.

"Oh, they're stable," he said. He read me the numbers.

Yes, everything was normal. Normal, that is, if you haven't just taken a shotgun to your face.

At kind of a loss for much else to ask, I said, "Is there an IV established?"

He told me there was an IV in the patient and running. I'm thinking, just how bad can this be? He must have missed and just taken off an ear or something. I walked over to see the patient.

He looked up at me and *damn*, he didn't miss. I was looking at a man that had no face left. Just two eyes, very cognizant, looking up from a deep pit of dripping hamburger meat. He had placed the shotgun under his chin when he fired the weapon. The mistake he made in trying to commit suicide was he leaned his head back when he pushed his thumb on the trigger. The effect was, he blew the lower part of his face off but it didn't go up into his head and brain, which would have killed him.

His lower jaw was gone. I mean *gone*. What was left of his nose was two small little flaps of skin where it split up the middle. The right side of his nose was a piece of skin stuck to what was left of his cheek under his right eye. Just a small little fragment of what was part of his left nose was just dangling dripping blood. From his cheek bones, which could be seen, down was mangled meat oozing blood at a slow but steady rate from everywhere. The blast had removed all the skin all the way over to his ears down to the top of his throat. What skin was left was sagging down, making finding landmarks in his neck impossible.

Now I know why everybody was just looking at him without doing anything. Oscar was alert. He was breathing without a problem. Well, if you consider not having a normal, recognizable, stable airway no problem, then yeah. Occasionally, he would hack a spray of blood out from wherever his windpipe was. But, other than that, he was breathing in and out and keeping good oxygen saturations going. Amazing. So, what was there to do?

Everything in your mind screamed this man needed to be intubated. But where? It was impossible to ascertain where his trachea was. I thought about poking around with a hemostat to find the hole the air was going in and coming out of. But really? We needed to medicate him and attempt to put in a breathing tube. But I knew, just looking at him, that this was going to be a very risky maneuver and probably not very successful. Not in the dark of his front yard in the middle of the night. His breathing was the only way that you could determine where his windpipe was. As soon as we turn him over on his back, he's going to drown in his own blood. How are we going to transport this patient? This was a conundrum.

There were times when you could do that one heroic maneuver with an advanced procedure and save a person's life. I've always said that there is a fine line between bravery and stupidity. The deciding factor is generally whether or not it was successful. Like if you jump from one rooftop to another rooftop. If you make it, it was brave but if you didn't, it was stupid. The most heroic part of bravery is knowing when not to try. In this case, he was sustaining his own airway, such that it was, and I determined it to be wiser to delay for a more optimum environment. Especially, because we could.

I looked at Mike, who looked at me. We both had the same look. What in the hell were we going to do. The ground crew were all looking at us as the flight crew who was supposed to know our stuff. They all must have been interested in what the flight nurse is going to come up with that they hadn't already thought of. My mind was racing.

"What's his blood pressure?" I asked, stalling for time to think.

"126 over 84," someone said.

Well, that was good. Damn it. That didn't give me much time to think. I felt like there was more that I should be doing but was damned to know what it was. I looked at Oscar looking at me. I knelt down to him.

"Do you feel like you're breathing okay?" I asked him in a loud voice, feeling somehow like he should at least be deafened somewhat. It freaked me out a little when he immediately nodded his head. Shit, this guy was completely lucid. Hell, Oscar was probably the calmest person out here right now. He was just unemotional. It made me pause.

"You think if you stay like this, in this position, you can breathe okay for a while?" I asked the rational eyes looking at me from a horror movie.

Again, he immediately nodded yes. It was just freaky as hell talking to a man with no face.

I stood up and looked around. All eyes were on me. "Let's just put him on a backboard in the position he's already in and transport him like that." I said. Surprisingly, my voice is decisive and direct. Like, "Hey, I've done these a thousand times, no problem."

"Okay," the captain said. "You heard him. Let's go."

"How are you going to secure him in the aircraft?" the captain asked.

With an air of authority now, I said, "Just like anyone else. We'll just put the belts across his back. That's all."

"You're going to Scottsdale Osborn, right?" the captain confirmed.

"Yes," I answered. "Can you give them a heads up? I don't know how busy I'm going to be once we lift. We should only be about five to ten minutes."

He nodded his agreement. We walked over to the aircraft carrying the patient on the longboard, with him on his belly holding his torso up on his elbows. Matt's face, watching us come up, was priceless. We slid him into place and secured the seatbelts around him. Ordinarily, I would put everyone on oxygen by face mask for the flight, as we were going up in altitude. But, in order to put on a face mask, you have to have a face. Thankfully, Oscar was oxygenating just fine, so it wasn't necessary.

I asked him how he was doing, and he nodded, indicating he was okay. Again, just freaky. Mike got in and hung the IV bag up and secured the monitor. After I secured the door, I came around and got in. Mike was busy putting down every towel and dressing he could find under the man's face to try to catch as much blood as possible from getting all over the place. His hamburger-meat face was oozing and dripping about as fast as our wide-open IV was running in.

"Good to go," I told Matt.

"Coming up," he replied. Off to Scottsdale Osborn trauma center.

Other than all the blood draining out of him, he was doing pretty well. Vital signs were holding stable and he was staying very alert. While en route Mike slipped in another IV, just so we had two good IVs running. This patient was going to need the fluids as well as plenty of IV access for drugs.

As we were flying along, I was looking at him. He was just

staring at the back bulkhead of the helicopter. It's said that the eyes are the windows of the soul. If that is the case, his soul looked extremely disturbed. Dark, deep, and lost. And with his eyes being the only thing left to his face, made it all the more pronounced.

When you have an injury, I find that the closer it is to the brain, the more intense the pain seems to be. That's why toothaches seem to be concentrated. That being said, this guy has to be in excruciating pain. But he hasn't indicated it. Then I thought, how was he supposed to without being able to talk or even scream.

I got as close as I dared to his faceless eyes and called out, "Are you in a lot of pain?"

Just as I said that, the thought crossed my mind: what a stupid question! Of course, he is.

The first time I actually saw definite emotion from him, he looked at me and started blinking rapidly.

"I'm going to give you something for it!" I yelled. "You think you can stay awake and in this position?"

Again, his eyes started blinking vehemently.

I wanted to do all that I could for this poor soul, but I was concerned about giving him something and having him relax and compromise his position and ability to maintain his airway and breathing. I pulled out my narcotics bag and grabbed what I thought would do the best. We carry a few different kinds of narcotics. I was drawing up the dose and thought about it. I drew up the maximum amount I'm allowed to give per protocol. I thought I was not really going to be able to give this patient so much with this injury, that it was going to get him comfortable enough to nod off. I mean, let's be real. His face is ripped off.

Once I gave it to him, his eyes go back to the concentrated stare. A couple minutes later, I asked if it helped. He blinked a couple of times, slower, for a gentle, yes, thank you.

The look on the faces of the trauma team was not that much different than the look on Matt's face as we were coming up to the helicopter. I don't think they've ever had a patient brought into the trauma room in a prone position before. Plus, the first sight of this man's missing face was insanely shocking. There was an unusual pause when we first came in. Then, suddenly, everyone snapped out of it and got to work. I shouted out a report as usual and then finished with my customary, "Any questions?"

"Yeah," the anesthesiologist spoke up. "Why didn't you intubate?"

"He's alert and maintaining an airway," I answered. "He's saturating well. I wanted to get him here, in the light, in a controlled environment before attempting that." The facial expression of the anesthesiologist indicated he understood that reasoning.

The trauma surgeon got down in front of the guy and talked to him for a minute, then stood up. "Let's get him intubated."

Oh, I couldn't wait to see how they're going to do this. *This* was a learning experience.

"Okay," the anesthesiologist said to the team. "I'm going to give him a sedative, then we'll turn him over before the paralytic."

Oh, I thought. I don't know if that's a good idea. But what do I know, I'm just a flight nurse.

He gave the sedative and then waited a few seconds for it to kick in. Oscar started to drift away, you could see it in his eyes. I was already well away from the action, but I actually took a couple more steps back in anticipation.

Once it was obvious the sedative had taken effect, the anesthesiologist said, "Okay, let's turn him over."

About five people in the team stepped up to roll Oscar over. I wondered why the anesthesiologist didn't ascertain exactly where the windpipe was before attempting this while Oscar was still breathing well. But, again, I'm not the expert here.

As soon as they rolled him over, all hell broke loose. Even with all the sedatives on board, Oscar came alive and started fighting and struggling, gasping and hacking. He was spewing blood like a whale; "Chimney's afire!" So hard and forcefully, the geyser was actually reaching the ceiling. There was blood everywhere. All over every person standing there, on the surgical lamp over the bed, the ceiling, all of the trays sitting close by. Everywhere. I'm glad I took a couple of precautionary steps back. I was well out of the line of fire.

"Give him the paralytic!" the trauma surgeon was exclaiming. "Give it now!"

The wide-eyed anesthesiologist was quickly grabbing IV tubing and shoving a syringe in and pushing. The flopping, blood-spewing fish continued for what seemed like minutes but was actually only seconds longer. Then, briefly, his body just went limp. People were still holding down his arms and legs when the anesthesiologist started to locate Oscar's trachea. Splattered in blood, and with his gloved hands fishing around in the shredded beef that was the man's throat, he desperately looked for a hole to put the breathing tube in. Oscar's present anatomy was not lending any clear clues to identify any discernable structures. This was all just a crap shoot.

Someone called out that his oxygen saturation was dropping. That just intensified the urgency to find the right hole. There was no "bagging" this guy. Even if you could get the mask over the right spot, there was no way to seal the mask to force air into the hole. This situation was getting dire. Just as the heart rate started to follow the oxygen saturation on a downward spiral, the anesthesiologist found what he thought might be the windpipe. He clamped the edge of it with a hemostat, held it taut, and pushed an endotracheal tube into the hole. He filled the balloon on the end of it and had someone bag the tube while he listened for lung sounds. The room is absolutely quiet. You couldn't even hear anyone else breath but you could almost hear everyone's heartbeat. It seemed like forever while he listened, then suddenly he stood up.

"We're in," he exhaled to everyone's relief.

Now that the intubation tube was in and semi-secured, everything was about what else could be done for this patient. Physiologically, he was stable. But how do you repair a face that was no longer there to repair.

Well, first things first. Take care of priorities. First of all, Oscar blew away his vocal cords in the blast. So, the balloon on the end of the endotracheal breathing tube that holds it in place by not coming past the vocal cords was no longer effective. They would have to secure the tube by another means. Mike and I felt we'd seen enough so we left as they started to suture in the breathing tube to what was left of Oscar's windpipe. They already started hanging blood to replace what he'd lost and the surgeon was discussing how to stop the bleeding.

"Well, that's a save," I said to Mike and Matt as we headed to the elevators to go up to the helipad. In emergency medical service, we see so many tragic events it's hard to imagine how something like this could be taken as just another call. But over time, it becomes just the nature of the business and you get used to it. Though in all honesty, it should never be anything that someone could get used to. But we have to and we often use humor to deal with it.

"Yeah," Mike added. "But what a mess. It's going to take hours to clean up the aircraft."

Blood had gotten everywhere. Even with the towels and pads, there was so much blood that it had drained down below the stretcher, onto the wall, the floor, some on the side of our bags, the monitor. Everywhere.

"So," Matt inquired, "are we down for clean up?" He needed to know when he called dispatch to clear from the hospital. Otherwise, it was possible to get another call immediately. This way they knew we needed to get back to base and have some time to get ready again.

"Oh yeah," Mike said, "we're down for now."

I am okay with that, because, to be honest, this was going to be one hell of a chart to write. Not that we did that much but explaining *why* we didn't do that much. This was an interesting call, a real learning experience. I just didn't want to have to answer to anybody on what we did and why. With this call, especially.

On the ride back to base, I found myself preoccupied thinking about Oscar. This was not the first attempted suicide I'd been called on. However, this was the first one I thought about the circumstances after the call. Whatever pushed Oscar to elect this course of action at this time? Whether it was a jilted lover, a faulty marriage, financial devastation, a failing business, a psychological disorder, or even a terminal, painful illness, I don't know. The reasons abound. But now, on top of whatever drove him to this end, he would have several surgeries, months of pain, permanent disfigurement, probably years of therapy, physical and phycological. Not to mention the cost. Some medical insurances will not cover self-inflicted injuries. All in all, it was going to be a long and difficult road added to the original reason. I felt for Oscar. I could never possibly put myself into the mind of another person. I would never tell someone, "I know how you feel." But that didn't stop me from feeling empathy for this single individual that I would have never known about if it was not for this call. I have to admit, I felt overwhelming sadness for this person I'd never met.

This was a pretty good time to take account of all of the troubles in my life and be thankful. One of the perks to this job; it'll make you appreciate your life. If you'll take the time to use it.

Chapter 15
DROWNED IN THE MOMENT

The crews that I worked with all had their own individual personalities. It was a wide range of personalities too. Most of them were class A personalities and more or less had to be. In this business, you had to be decisive, direct, determined, and sure of yourself. Not full of yourself but sure of yourself. There is very much a difference between the two distinctions.

Everyone had their opinions about everything, but when it came to work, everyone left their opinions at the door. It dawned on me, in later years, the kind of people I was privileged to work with in this career. They were not just top notch in what they did, they were really some of the best people I would ever hope to know. They weren't merely colleagues, I considered them family. The company was small enough in the early years that you got to know your crew members, their significant others, their kids, hell, even their pets.

One very memorable call early on when we started the company was with Leslie. We were still very much the new kids on the block and, to that end, we were very cautious about how we came across to the ground crews and the public in general. Leslie was sometimes my paramedic. She was a stocky lady in her early thirties, determined and extremely competent in her profession. She wore John Denver-type glasses; her hair was close cropped and her walk was not feminine. She didn't mix words either. She was as pleasant as a school teacher but just as direct.

Our radios came alive with a scramble to a place not very far from us. Like I said, this was in the early years, not long after I started with NAAA. About six months. Long enough to get comfortable in my job and secure with my performance. Coffey was the pilot-in-command for this shift. That always made things interesting because if you got a call, Coffey was entertaining. It was just his personality.

"Native 1 scramble, Native 1 scramble, Baseline and Gilbert for a pediatric drowning," the radio called out.

At this point, we hadn't even come up with the term Charlie Foxtrot, but even then, I knew we were going to walk into one. Almost anytime it had to do with a child, people on scene would get excited—and the more serious, the more excited. If the kid was really critical … forget about it.

We were over to the scene in no time flat. You could hear the tension in the voice of the firefighter giving us landing instructions. Especially when he felt the need to tell us to, "Stay hot."

That was our common practice and they knew that. There was no need to tell us unless you were excited about it. When they would say that, it generally meant they were going to run the patient out to us as soon as we landed. Thinking that was going to speed things up. Completely missing the fact that they needed to be escorted into the landing zone, at least under the rotor disk, or the turning blades, by a flight crew member. Not to mention the fact that I still needed to get some kind of report to tell the doctor at the emergency room. You can't just throw us some kid and say, "Take off!"

But that was just what we were seeing as we were making our descent. A responder holding a small child doing piss poor compressions while another was trying to bag the little kid in his arms. One of the responders was off to the side holding the monitor and the captain next to them on the radio. These guys were a discombobulated mess. *Man*, I thought, *this is going to be ugly*. Leslie was on the side of the helicopter facing away from them as we were coming down.

I keyed up the mic, "Get ready, sis, this is going to be nuts."

They were already making their way to the aircraft before Coffey was even settled enough to take his hands off the controls. Hell, they were almost already at the door before I could get out.

Under the wind and noise of the engine and thumping rotor blades, I screamed, "What's up?"

"Two-year-old girl found at the bottom of the pool!" the captain yelled. "Tried to intubate twice already without success. CPR since we got here. You guys need to go."

There was no IV established, that was obvious. The way they were holding the limp child, CPR was anything but effective. The monitor was showing a flatline heart rate. If this kid had any chance for survival, she needed a breathing tube. She didn't need a whole emergency department, she needed decent respirations. Especially in pediatric patients, breathing is everything.

The medic put the girl on our gurney that was angled out slightly and continued doing CPR.

"She needs to be intubated!" I said loud enough to be heard over the rotor noise.

"You need to go!" screamed the fire captain.

Leslie had all the intubation equipment out and ready to go. She handed me the appropriate sized laryngoscope and was preparing the elastic tubes of the appropriate sizes to give me when needed.

"You need to go!" screamed the fire captain, again.

I put the blade of the scope in the mouth of the small child and down her throat. Lifting just right, the vocal cords were easily seen. What was so hard about that? I took the 4.5 endotracheal tube Leslie handed me and slipped it right through the cords without a problem. Prefect, textbook. Leslie put the ambu bag on the end of the tube and applied a couple of squeezes. The medic continued to do CPR. Intubation was so quick and easy that he never even stopped while I was tubing. As Leslie bagged a couple of times, water came up the tube.

"It's not in the right place!" the captain shouted. He reached over and grabbed the tube and pulled it out. Before I even knew what was happening, or could stop it, the tube was out. "You need to go!" he screamed yet again.

The medic doing compressions was at it hot and heavy. He was looking at the captain and glaring at me.

The tube was in, damn it! Normally, when you miss the trachea and inadvertently intubate the esophagus, when you bag the patient, you'll get stomach contents up through the tube. Sometimes it may look like water and that is one of the signs that you're not in the right place, so you pull the tube out and start again. But not in this case. This child had just drowned. What do you expect was going to come up out of the tube? Her lungs were full of water. But that was what the captain was seeing and thought the tube was misplaced. I wondered how many times they actually successfully intubated this kid and after bagging water out, pulled the tube, thinking it was in the wrong place. Well, the only thing this kid needed right now was a patent, stable airway that can force air past the water. She needed to be intubated.

"Let's do it again," I told Leslie, who was already handing me the scope.

"You get going!" the captain screamed at me. "Or so help me God, I will punch you out."

I'd never been assaulted while doing my job by a fellow scene crew member before. I remember thinking, *This is an interesting development.* I wasn't sure how I felt because there wasn't time to concern myself about it. Whatever the case, this patient needed to be intubated now. She didn't need to go, she needed to breathe. Feeling like a discussion at this point was futile and time wasting, I ignored the captain and continued on. I put the scope back down the child's throat, concentrating on what I was doing. I could feel the piercing stare of the captain on my head and was waiting for a reaction from him.

The tube went in again without a problem. I didn't even need to listen to lung sounds, I was sure of the placement. Leslie started to bag the tube again, and, again, water came up.

"You see, it's not in!" the captain hollered again. He reached up to grab the tube.

I quickly blocked his reach to the tube, preventing him from pulling it out.

"Leave it and we'll go!" I loudly told him under the rotor blades.

He gave me a death glare. He was pissed. "Well, go then!" he screamed at me. "You should have been gone fifteen minutes ago!"

A perfect example of time distortion in these situations. I

don't know if he meant it or it was just an exaggeration. But, in fact, our skids had only touched down less than two minutes before. All this happened in that short amount of time.

Leslie was already in the aircraft and bagging the child. I took over compressions from the medic so they could leave the landing zone. As soon as they were clear, Leslie took over compressions so I could belt in the child, secure the door, and get in myself. As soon as I was in, I told Coffey we were ready to go. Instantly, the aircraft lifted and we were off.

In all honesty, this child didn't look viable, especially after being down for so long. But children are remarkably resilient and can bounce back from disastrous events. We felt the need to keep trying until all possibilities were exhausted.

While taking off, I got an IV kit out and looked for a site. Leslie was doing fine with compressions and occasionally bagging as necessary. Surprisingly, the little girl had a vein I was able to stick right away and I secured the IV and started to prepare resuscitation drugs.

As I was preparing an amp of Epinephrine, I heard a knocking on the door. About the same time, Coffey came over the intercom, "You guys hear that?"

"Yeah," I replied. "What is it?"

"I'm not sure," Coffey said. "Are all the seatbelts in?"

Damn it. I looked and realized, in all the chaos, I inadvertently left a seatbelt hanging out. This was a short little two-year-old girl that didn't need all the belts to secure her. Now that belt was beating the hell out of Little Girl's side as we flew through the air at over a hundred and twenty miles an hour. We didn't have a choice. We had to set down and put the seatbelt back in the helicopter before it caused irreparable damage to the aircraft. Not what we needed right now. Luckily, we were over an open field at the time and Coffey set the aircraft down. I jumped out and got the seatbelt put back in the aircraft. The buckle had left a few marks on the side but nothing other than cosmetic damage. Quickly, we were back on our way.

Scottsdale Osborn Hospital was the closest facility to us at the time. Not a pediatric facility, but that didn't matter. We needed to be in a hospital to attempt to get her stabilized. She had been down for an unknown amount of time and was showing no signs of life. Pupils were fixed and dilated from the time I saw her, and they never changed. During transport, Coffey had alerted the ground crew where we were going so they could tell the parents where to meet us. This was one of the few times when we had a hot off-load. We didn't wait to shut down the helicopter. We jumped out and unloaded her and took her straight in.

Not to my surprise, the trauma team only continued resuscitation efforts for a few more minutes before pronouncing her dead. With all the efforts, drugs, and procedures we had performed, no changes in life signs were ever noted. This was not a save. And this was one that I wished in every way could have been.

Also, not to my surprise, we were notified immediately upon returning to base that we had a complaint against us. Well, not exactly us. Me. The fire captain was livid. He wanted a debrief with his medical control doctor and ours. Medical control are the doctors that give us our standing orders and supervise and critique our efforts. Medical control is also another name for the doctors that are in charge of our individual programs. Whose license we work under.

In other words, I was being called out.

When Coffey heard about this, he got a little annoyed to say the least. He was able to hear the exchange between the captain and me, even under the din of the helicopter.

He told me, "I was about to shut off the aircraft and come around to see what the captain had to say to me."

All joking aside, no one wanted to piss off Coffey. I was humbled that he had my back the whole way. He insisted on being at any conference pertaining to this incident.

Two days later I was informed to be at the fire station conference room for a meeting between all parties involved. There was the fire captain, the medic doing the compressions, their medical control doctor, our medical control doctor, Coffey, and myself. The entire scenario was laid out, first from the captain's point of view and then my side of the story. When all was said and done, both doctors agreed that I acted professionally and appropriately, even adding that under the distress of the situation, I had acted exactly the way they would have in the same instance. My actions were not the inappropriate ones.

Out of the heat of the moment and under the clear analytical light of hindsight, both the captain and the medic could see the obvious rationale of my actions. The captain sincerely apologized for his response at the scene. I harbored no ill will towards him or the medic. I understood the gravity of the situation and how heavily it can weigh on a person at the time. Grave situations involving kids are highly charged and very emotional. That was the reason I worked diligently to keep my emotions in check during any such scene calls. Emotions don't allow you to think with a clear head. And that's imperative, especially in the most trying of times.

Unexpectantly, in future scene calls with this particular

captain, he was incredibly friendly and courteous to me, very respectful. We even talked and joked with each other on scene like old friends. Funny, this business is.

Chapter 16
THE ANTLER GUY

Chad was my most frequent partner in the early years of NAAA. Because of the way schedules were put together, you didn't always get the same partner. More often than not, however, Chad would be with me. We tried to make it that way. I loved it. Chad was ten years younger than I was. He was a superb paramedic, we worked well together from the very start; we had a good chemistry. More than that, he was vastly entertaining. He had an uncanny resemblance to Jim Carrey, and when he wanted to, could look and act just like him. His wit and humor were just as sharp, especially when he did Fire Marshall Bill from the *In Living Color* comedy show.

In those days, Chad and I spent a lot of time killing time. Frisbee on the tarmac, even walking into Rick's office and just sitting on the couch, playing cards. Rick would look up from his desk and ask what we were doing. We'd casually look at him and remark, "Well, you said you had an open-door policy. It was open, so we thought we'd just come in and sit with you awhile." He was not amused with the humor and promptly commanded us to leave.

One night we were scrambled to Superior, Arizona, for a

motor vehicle that had gone over a cliff. They wanted us to stage and standby at the tiny airport that was just outside of Superior, out in the middle of nowhere with nothing around for miles. It was February and one of the few times it was freezing cold in Arizona. Before we landed, we found out that they were still trying to just get to the crashed vehicle. It was lodged about seventy-five feet down the side of a cliff and being held by the trees. They were unsure of any injuries at this time. So, it was going to take a while before they would need us. When we landed, Matt went on and shut down the aircraft.

It didn't take long for the cold to permeate the aircraft. I would rarely bring a jacket on a call. It would just be bulky and get in the way in an area you didn't have much room in to begin with. When I was out working on a patient, I didn't think about the cold so it didn't matter to me. Such as it was this night. After a while, however, I started to regret that decision. One of my early learning experiences was *always have a jacket in the cargo hold*. The temperature hovered just above freezing at about thirty-four degrees.

Thankfully, we had Chad. About fifteen minutes of sitting there talking about normal everyday stuff, the cold really started to sink in. Then Chad got started. First, he went into a Fire Marshall Bill monologue. Then he started telling jokes. How this guy could remember so many jokes was beyond me. Then he'd go into another routine from some movie comedy like *Major Payne,* and he'd do it to perfection. It was non-stop. Matt and I would get to laughing so hard we actually had to get out of the aircraft to calm down and cool off. I'd get out laughing and damn if Chad wouldn't get out right behind us and continue on. It got to where my sides were hurting.

Two hours passed without us even knowing it when

the radio clicked on. "Native 1, you can stand down. You're cancelled. You can return to base."

We all looked down at our watches and realized how long we'd been stranded there and for no reason. Just to get cancelled. We looked up at each other and then Chad went into another character that played out our situation perfectly. We were off rolling again, couldn't stop. We didn't even care why we were cancelled.

It took minutes for Matt to compose himself enough to fire up the bird.

"Cranking the shit out of it!" he blurted out.

Now that line had Chad barking out an unstoppable laugh. It was a long, freezing cold, miserable, remarkably fun night.

Months later, I was with Chad again and it was just after midnight. We were sitting in the dispatch office when a call came in. After a second or two, the dispatcher looked at us and twirled his finger in the air.

It was for a motor vehicle versus a pedestrian. Most of the time, pedestrians don't fare well when they tangle with a moving vehicle. It was on the entrance ramp to Interstate 10, far south of us in Maricopa. EMS was on the way but not there yet. They wanted us to go on and launch to the scene. We obliged them immediately. If they got there and it was nothing, they'd cancel en route. But it's pretty rare that a pedestrian can get struck by a motor vehicle and not sustain an injury; a reasonably significant injury, actually often death. After a while going to scene calls, even caring people that got into this profession to help other people in a crisis, become so used to tragedy that it becomes expected and routine. What kind of mess is this going to be, I wondered?

Halfway down to the scene we were notified that they

were indeed going to transport the patient, which meant he was injured. During our orbit over the scene, I saw several emergency vehicles with their lights flashing and a large pick-up truck down the entrance ramp from the overpass intersection. The truck was one of those raised up, big tired, monster-truck looking pick-ups, just not nearly as big as the show vehicles. All the people were standing in a spot midway up the ramp, just standing around a guy sitting on the curb. We landed on part of the overpass that had been blocked off for us. Chad and I got out and walked down to the scene. Chad went over to the patient as I was met on the way by the paramedic.

He was giving me report that this guy was one of those homeless folks that you see sometimes at the intersections panhandling. It's late, he's been drinking, and he was sitting on the curb when the truck came around and struck him. The driver of the truck was being tested for possible DUI by the Highway Patrol officers. The driver was unharmed. Minimal damage to the truck except for the front bumper that obviously struck the victim.

Unknown if the patient sustained a loss of consciousness, the paramedic reported, but he was conscious by the time the driver got back to see if he was okay.

"He's pretty drunk," the paramedic stated. "And he won't let us do much. He's not combative, just really uncooperative."

The paramedic stopped for a moment. Looked at me and said, "He really needs to be flown to a trauma center."

I could see he was trying not to laugh. He looked down, shaking his head. Composed, he looked back up at me, "Yeah, he needs to go." Unable to restrain it anymore, he smiled.

"The only information I've been able to get from him is that his name is Jim." That was about all the paramedic could give me.

I was looking at the patient talking to Chad. From my angle, I could just see a profile view of the left side of his head. Everything looked about normal, except for flashing red and blue lights reflecting off his head. I looked back at the paramedic perplexed.

After getting the report, I walked up to Jim sitting on the curb. He turned to look at me face on. That night I should have won an Academy Award for maintaining the completely concerned, professional expression I displayed just then. Now I understood the smile on the paramedic's face.

My partner and another medic were trying, unsuccessfully, to put a neck collar on the guy. He was not cooperating with the procedure. He was having nothing to do with it. Alcohol intoxication easily explained his behavior. I walked up and knelt down in front of Jim at a safe distance that didn't seem intrusive. I didn't want to do anything that was going to put the man on the defensive. I was trying not to start grinning. The sight in front of me was tragically hilarious.

"Hi. Jim is it?" I asked to start a dialog with him. "I'm a nurse on the helicopter. I'm here to give you assistance. Do you know what happened tonight?"

"Yeah," he answered sluggishly. "I think I was hit by a truck."

"Yeah, you were." I told him calmly.

Every time he turned his head to look at what was going on, it got a little harder to maintain my composure. You have to understand. I'm kneeling down, talking to a guy who was completely coherent, except for the obvious alcohol intoxication. He was alert, responsive, attentive to all the fuss that was being made about him right then. He was turning his head from side to side, looking at all the people standing around him.

He was moving freely and he had an eight-inch-long, three-inch-wide piece of plastic bumper from the truck sticking out of the right side of his head like some antler on a moose. It was a dark, metallic-green plastic piece from the front part of the truck that was well embedded in Jim's skull. It was solidly stuck there. Every time he moved his head, the antler moved with it just like it had always been there. I was pretty sure old Jim didn't have a clue that it was there or how it looked. Other than really freaky, it was fucking hysterical. It made me think of when someone sees or hears something that's not right, they say: *they had a flag go up.* This was like the literal sense of the phrase. He had a flag sticking up out of his head. It's hard to explain why it seemed so funny except that it was not supposed to be there, in his head and he shouldn't have been so cognizant with it stuck there. When he moved his head, it didn't flop around or change position, it was part of him like an antler. It was so tight, he wasn't even bleeding.

"Jim," I continued, in the most soothing voice I could muster. "You were hit by a truck. And, well, right now you have a rather large piece of the bumper sticking out of your head. That's really not a good thing."

He looked at me. "Can't you just pull it out?"

"Well, Jim, no, we can't." I allowed a little time for his inebriated brain to process what I was telling him. "I'm not sure how deep the piece in your head is. I suspect it's probably into the brain and needs to be seen by a doctor." This was concerning to us, but there was nothing we could do here but transport him to a hospital for surgery.

He looked at me, trying to register what I'd said. He reached up to grab the piece. Suddenly, everybody jumped toward him. "No!" "Don't grab it!" "Stop!" The last thing we needed was for him to yank the thing out and have blood squirting across the roadway. If he even could pull it out.

I maintained my posture and position, "Hang on, Jim. Don't fool with it. It's okay for now, but don't take it out."

Slowly, his hand came back down. He looked around at all the people standing there. Every time he moved his head I just wanted to cry … in laughter. *It was just funny*. It was unnaturally freakish. That was the only way I could process it; as humorous.

Two of the people standing by us were police officers. Those were the two that drew Jim's attention the most.

"Am I going to be arrested?" he asked.

"No," I reassured him. "We just want to take you to the hospital to get you cared for. These guys have to make a report because you were injured. That's all. You're the victim here."

Finally, Jim consented to be taken to the hospital. "You gonna fly me in that helicopter?"

"Yeah," I replied. "We're some ways from the hospital and you need to be seen pretty quickly. Are you going to be okay with that?"

He took a moment and then nodded. Antler and all.

"Now, we're going to have to put a neck collar on and strap you down on the board," I prepared him. "That's just what we have to do to secure you in the aircraft. Plus, if we walk in to the hospital without the neck collar, the doctor will chew us out. Can you help us out and let us do that?"

He nodded again. Then, surprisingly, he stood up and sat on the longboard that was placed next to him some time ago. He allowed Chad and the other medic to put the neck collar on without resistance of any kind. Then, he just laid back on the backboard and let them strap him down. Actually, a very cordial gentleman when you could get him to agree.

"I need to start an IV on you," I told him, expecting a stern decline. "So I can give you some drugs. Something for the pain. Are you okay with that?"

He shrugged and just laid there. I primed the IV tubing while Chad easily popped in an IV in his left arm. No reaction from Jim whatsoever. I gave him some pain medication and an antiemetic. While in flight, Chad and I worked together to pad and wrap a dressing around the antler base. Not that it was bleeding much at all, more to just stabilize it. Plus, it really seemed like the thing to do.

We flew him to the closest trauma center at Maricopa County Medical Center. The trauma teams at MCMC are some of the finest you'll find anywhere. The hospital sits right in the center of downtown Phoenix on the more impoverished side of the city. A result of which is that they see more volume of devastating traumas than some other trauma units in town. They tend to get the worst of the worse and they tend to get them more often. Plus, the hospital harbors the only burn unit in the city, so traumas that involve burns tend to get routed to MCMC. They are also one of the only pediatric trauma units at this time. These folks see it all, all the time.

Being a teaching hospital, they have attending physicians watching over interns and first, second, third, and fourth year residents. All vying to get in there and get their hands dirty and show what they're made of. Not only are they incline to drill for different scenarios, but they get to practice often. Once you bring a patient into the room and step back, the patient disappears into the center of green scrub suits and white lab coats. There's very little they haven't encountered.

We rolled in with Jim on the flight gurney and lined him up with the trauma stretcher. I noticed for the briefest of moments everyone was motionless and silent. They were all taking in the picture of our perfectly normal acting, very cognizant patient with a bumper sticking out of his head, very calm and peaceful like. They all looked unusually stunned for a second.

There was more head scratching and lip pulling going on than anything else at this point. Jim was just lying there gazing up at them, looking like you would expect any person to look being stared at like an alien. He could not see the foreign object protruding from his skull like everyone else could. Then everyone got to work like normal. I got my chart signed and left.

Now, I was not insensitive to his plight. The fact that Chad and I were grinning ceaselessly did not mean that we were crude and unfeeling. We knew that this was a very serious situation. That piece of plastic was undoubtingly protruding into poor Jim's brain. How far, we didn't know. This could easily cause permanent brain damage and could even turn out to be fatal. This was very serious indeed.

We were not laughing *at* Jim or his inebriated state. In this job, you witness some very unusual sights. This was one of the oddest I'd ever encountered. You would see things happen that you would never think could happen. Or, that you would never think to think about happening. You could be upset by it, disturbed by it, or just laugh it off. That's why so many in this business get such a strange and morbid sense of humor. It's the nature of the job. You see things that are funny, like something you'd see in a cartoon, that are really not funny. They're tragic. So, humor is used to maintain sanity. It's really the only way you can continue to do this job. I have never seen or heard of anyone laughing at someone's tragedy. You would just find humor in some of the things you would see, and hope that they'd never happen to you. Looking at Jim with this enormous foreign body sticking out of his head was hard to look at and heartrending. We really did feel concern for him.

But we couldn't help it, that shit there was just funny.

"Well," I said on the way out, "that's a save."

Chad looked at me with that Jim Carrey quizzical look, "Uh, you think that's fair game?"

Oh yeah, the puns were already starting.

Chapter 17
OUT OF LIMITS

Before Native 5 opened and when I was still going to work at Williams-Gateway Airport, occasionally I'd pick up an over-time shift on the fixed-wing aircraft. Most of the time, the calls were a little more relaxed. It wasn't likely to have to respond to a scene call in an airplane. Not to say that they were going to be any less critical. Sometimes a patient would have to be transferred in an airplane because of the severity and equipment needed was more than a helicopter could handle. I've taken extremely critical patients on the fixed-wing often. The distance for fixed-wing calls was generally much greater, even with the added time going to and from the airport in an ambulance, it would be quicker than a helicopter to transport by airplane because they could cruise much faster over that expanse. But because the distance was farther, that meant that you were going to be spending more time with the patient. More time with the patient gave more time for things to go wrong. Airplanes could also be pressurized, as a result they could fly higher without exposing the patient to the unwanted detrimental effects of altitude. Something you couldn't do in a helicopter.

I liked an occasional shift on the airplane. With the right crew, it could be a lot of fun. There was always plenty of room to move around and you could stand up and stretch if you needed to. Not to mention, that you had at least four people helping load the patient. Two pilots and two medical crew. That was always a plus.

One night I was flying with Chad, who decided to pick up the shift also. A rare instance when both positions were not covered on the schedule. The pilots tonight would be Shawn as captain and John, his first officer. They were a good pair as they normally flew together on the same shifts. Even being relatively young, in his early thirties, the red-headed, light-skinned Shawn had been flying forever. He reminded me of a young Ron Howard from *Happy Days*. He started very young and had a lot of experience. He carried an air of confidence about him but was not especially arrogant. Shawn had a maturity to his youth but was youthful just the same.

John, on the other hand, was young, in his twenties, but you couldn't tell by the size of him. Big fella. Dark haired, jovial dude that was always into doing something physical while waiting for a call. Throwing a baseball or a Frisbee around with someone on the tarmac. Many a night we'd kill a few hours tossing the Frisbee back and forth with the multiple crews stationed there. Most of the first officers were young, new pilots. They didn't have to have a lot of time or expertise because they were always shadowed by an experienced captain on board. In fact, that's why most of them were here; to get flight time in and build their experience base.

It was always a pleasure to fly with these two guys and was partly the reason Chad and I decided to take the shift. They came on to cover the night shift. Chad and I had sat all day, watching a little TV, napping a little, and spending some time in the dispatch shack talking and watching video games. When Shawn and John came on, we went out together to the airplane to do our nightly brief. There was good-hearted banter intermixed with the necessary instructions and checks. John was always the one to get started joking, but when Chad got started, nobody could hold a candle to him. Before long, all of us were laughing and adding to the continuous humor. Even Shawn, who prided himself on keeping a straight face and attempting to maintain the air of "captain" of the ship, was cutting up. It seemed necessary to have someone keep the seriousness of the nature of our business readily in mind. But, with the four of us, familiar and seasoned with each other, we allowed ourselves to be jovial.

Later that night, our crew and the rotor crew were sitting in the greenroom in the hangar with the TV on. We weren't really watching it because conversations would get started. Commonly, it would take about an hour and a half, or more, to try to decide what program to watch or what video movie to put in. We would rarely ever just sit and watch quietly anyway.

The greenroom had an intercom system in it connected to the dispatch office. When the fixed-wing crew would get a call, it would be announced over that initially. It was late, but everyone was still up making sporadic and humorous commentary to the movie we were watching. You would hear a slight pop and a hiss in the intercom speaker when it was keyed, alerting you that dispatch was about to say something. It was enough to make everyone stop what they were doing, quiet down and listen. Then you'd hear our dispatcher deliver the message. Lifeguard 1, the designation for our aircraft, was being launched to San Carlos. With everyone there, our crew got up to the shouts of "Yeehaw," "Here we go," "Let's get it on," "Go to it, boys," and "Y'all be safe." Getting a call was always a reason to get excited because you were going to do something, earn your money, make money for the company. You were going to go do your job instead of sitting around. In the early years, when you're new, you wanted that. The four of us grabbed our stuff and headed out through the hangar to the awaiting Jetstream on the tarmac.

The report I received was that we were going to pick up a 380-pound male with acute ETOH poisoning. ETOH stands for Ethanol Alcohol. A nice way of saying, alcohol intoxication. In other words, we were going to get a very large drunk guy. This wouldn't be the first time I witnessed an alcohol overdose that, despite what you or the doctors do, progressed to multi-organ failure and death. So, this could be very serious. Most of the time, however, it was strictly precautionary. It was reported that he was not intubated and on a ventilator. That was almost always a good sign. Unless it needed to be done and hadn't been done yet.

San Carlos was a small Native American settlement far east of Phoenix with a small hospital servicing it. Easily a three-hour ambulance ride to the closest hospital in the Phoenix area. The hospital is so small and rural that they can easily become overwhelmed. Many times, walking into the emergency department in a small community was like coming into a situation that still needed emergent procedures done. It was not uncommon for small rural hospitals to lack the experience and equipment that bigger city hospitals have. Many times, these hospitals would prefer to have the more experienced flight crews come in and intubate or administer critical amounts of medications. Because of our experience and frequent exposure to these procedures, we were more comfortable with them and they were more comfortable with us doing them. Most of us would call it a "well-lit scene call" because about as much would be done as when we would land on a scene. We would never mention that to anyone because it would sound arrogant but it was truthful in some instances. With just a doctor and one nurse on duty, you generally had more help and more vital procedures done on a scene call with several firefighters and paramedics than you'd have here. Communities like this relied on aeromedical support for advanced equipment, assistance and rapid transport to a higher-level of care facility. Plus, with generally only one ambulance in the area, transporting by air kept that one ambulance available to the community when needed.

Coming into San Carlos, the airport is on top of a small mesa. The area is completely unsecured. The mesa is a flat, raised area within the community just up a winding road from the hospital. The landing strip had only about fifty percent of the runway lights operational, sporadically spaced along either edge. The rest of the lights had been busted out by rocks thrown at them for target practice. When you have such a small little community so isolated and distant from anything else, you get a lot of bored young people with nothing to do and nowhere to go. So, consequently, they have to devise their own form of entertainment.

When Chad and I walked into the emergency room, which was really a large area at the end of the hall with a desk, counter, and four beds, each surrounded with a drawn privacy curtain, we saw the doctor. I could hear the nurse behind one of the curtains talking to a patient.

The doctor stood up. "Hey, glad you're here. We have a

guy going down to Phoenix with elevated ETOH levels. Really needs to be seen."

The doctor was typical for this place. A relatively recent graduate of medical school, here to pay off some of his commitment to the government for loans. Indian reservations are generally on federal lands and, as such, acquire federal assistance. In this case, medical doctor coverage. You may be somewhat inexperienced when you get here, but that quickly changes when you're the sole provider in a diverse medical situation. Dealing with everything from premature labor, to extreme cases of diabetes, to some rather dramatic traumas. It's great experience.

Chad went in to see and assess the patient while I received report from the doctor.

"This is Rodney, he came in about four hours ago," the doctor went on, coming around the counter with the paperwork. "He's actually doing pretty good considering." He stopped there and handed me the lab report.

I looked down at the lab report, what caught my eye was the ETOH level. I looked up at the doctor. He looked at me with a glimmer in his eye, a slight grin and nodded.

"Is this correct?" I questioned.

"Yes," he answered. "It's been done twice."

"Impressive." That was all I could say.

This 380-pound, thirty-year-old male, who I could hear talking behind the curtain, had an ETOH level of 540, or what most people know as, 0.54. Where 0.08 is the legal limit, 0.16 you're generally pretty sloshed, 0.28 you're generally passed out, and 0.35 you're normally playing with death, unless you're an alcoholic. Yet this guy was 0.54. And, I could hear him talking. Yup, impressive.

"Has he been given anything?" I asked the doctor.

"No." He turned around to look at his paperwork on the counter. "We put in an IV. Well, I take that back. I did give him a couple of Tylenol for a headache and some Thiamine IV." He gave me a humorous glance. "But, that's about it. I just want him to go down to Phoenix to be watched. This is an unusual amount and could have devastating affects down the road."

I concurred. I still couldn't believe I was hearing this guy talking. Not only that, it was not even that slurred or disoriented. I couldn't wait to see him. All the time, in the back of my mind was the concern that this guy could suddenly succumb to the effects of such a high amount of alcohol and become comatose and have to be intubated. This was a big fella, he was not going to be easy to intubate if needed.

I stepped behind the curtain and saw this very round gentleman happily sitting up in the middle of the bed with a gigantic, inebriated grin on his face. He was one happy soul. What was fascinating to me was his relative clarity of voice, his focus and attention to his environment, and his noticeable lack of wobble. This was not a tall guy. His 380-pound mass was contained in about five-feet six-inches of framework. He was round and had absolutely no neck. In fact, his head appeared to be below his shoulders. Again, it crossed my mind that this guy would be incredibly difficult to intubate if I had to. *Please, don't let me have to.*

"Hello," I said to him.

"Heeellllooo," he responded. Grinning ear to ear.

I looked at the nurse and she smiled at me. No doubt glad I was here and she was transferring care to me. I looked at Chad, he was smiling also, humored by the cheerful patient sitting in the bed, completely cooperative with everything he was doing. Chad was so amused, he quietly laughed while he tried to keep up with the ecstatic guy's movements long enough to get the monitor applied. The patient was very animated and very friendly. Get close enough and he'd give you a kiss. Very friendly.

"Can you tell me how much you've had to drink today?" I asked him, expecting the old "two-beer" answer. I don't care how drunk somebody is, when you ask them how much they've had to drink, it's always, "Two beers."

"Well," he stopped to contemplate. It was almost comical to see how fast he went from hilarious to serious thought. "Let's see. I had about a fifth of vodka this morning, then me and a buddy was drinking on a half-gallon of Wild Turkey, then we had a six pack. No, a 12-pack. Then, tonight, had some more vodka and another six-pack. And, about four shots of tequila." He looked up at me with a large smile of pride. "I think that's about all."

While he was calm, momentarily deep in thought, Chad was able to get the blood pressure cuff on.

"Oh," the guy popped out. "I forgot, had a pint of rum too. Spiced rum. Good stuff. You don't have any, do you?"

I shook my head. "No, I don't think we carry that." I was astonished Rodney was able to remember everything as well as he did.

"Can we stop and get some?" He looked at me. He wasn't joking now. His gaze showed me it was a serious question.

Chad was unable to suppress his laugh. The nurse was laughing as she walked away.

"No," I answered and couldn't help but smile too. "I don't think so. Not on the way, anyhow."

"Oh, shoot," he mumbled.

With our stretcher close to the bed, Chad asked him if he thought he could scoot over. Before anyone could take a breath, Rodney pushed himself to the end of the bed and stood up. Suddenly, both Chad and I jumped to catch him. But to our total surprise, he very steadily took one step up to the stretcher and climbed on. Absolutely no wobble whatsoever. There was no way his ETOH was 540. I went back to look at the first original lab value that they didn't believe and prompted a repeat blood draw. It was 590 then. Incredible!

We strapped him onto to flight stretcher with the three seatbelts that just barely fit around his gargantuan girth after a little manipulation. I thanked the nurse and doctor, and they gave me a "good luck" thumbs up on the way out. As we walked down the hall, our fella was just a happy little bird, singing and laughing all the way out, waving at everyone there as we passed.

We got to the aircraft and had to envision sliding Rodney up the ramp, through the doors and into the stretcher block. The Jetstream was reasonably high off the ground and it had the normal passenger-width door. Our gleeful patient was almost as wide as he was tall. Thankfully, not only did we have four in our team but we also had the two crewmembers from the ambulance to assist. Jolly ol' Rodney suggested letting him walk onto the plane, but I couldn't have, in good conscious, permitted that. There would be no way to explain why I allowed that if anything were to happen. Not to mention, if he did faulter on the way up, who was going to attempt to catch him? Nope, we were going to have to slide him up the ramp and through the doors using brute force. It actually went along rather well, despite him laughing and joking all the way, making it more difficult, because we were all giggling while grunting.

Once Shawn had gotten the aircraft fired up and with us all secured and ready, he announced we were rolling. The Jetstream built up speed rapidly. About at the end of the runway, I felt Shawn pull the nose of the airplane up sharply to lift. Maybe, a little sharper than usual, but it had been a while since I'd ridden with him. I felt a slight jolt as we were lifting off the ground. But I didn't pay it any mind.

Almost immediately our happy little patient was looking out the window and nodding off. All I could think was, just don't become unresponsive and need intervention. I noticed Chad was keeping a good look at him for the same reason. That helped put me at ease. Knowing that, in all the fun, he was just as concerned as I was. I heard the whine of the flap motors whirl, retracting the flaps as we continued to climb to altitude. All was good and we had about a forty-minute flight to Phoenix. Plenty of time to complete the chart and relax.

It caught my eye the amount of movement going on in the cockpit. Normally, by this time, it was pretty quiet up there. All you'd see were glowing lights. Shortly, I saw John turn around and look at me, then he motioned for me to come up. This was unusual and had my curiosity stirred. I made my way up to the cockpit. I braced myself in the threshold between the cabin and cockpit in case of air pockets as we were still slowly climbing to cruise altitude. I glanced at the instrumentation on the dash to see if there was anything amiss. I'm no pilot, but I've spent enough time in the cockpit of various aircraft to know what to look for and get a feel for the condition of the flight. Everything looked pretty nominal. Except, the landing gear lights were still green. They hadn't been retracted yet.

Shawn slipped his headset off one ear and I did the same. He looked up at me with an obvious expression of concern in the reflective glow of the dash lights.

"How's everything going back there?" he asked. Which had me wondering because this had never been asked before.

"Fine," I responded. "The guys doing okay." I turned to look back at the patient. "He's snoring right now." I turned back around and looked at Shawn, "Why?"

"Did you feel a bump when we were taking off?"

I thought about it for a moment. "Uh, well, yeah, kind of."

"Well," he hesitated, "we hit a rock, a big rock and something else at the end of the runway. It looked like a railroad tie or something like that. I was committed to the take-off by the time we saw them, so I pulled up hoping to miss them. But we didn't. We tapped them coming off. I don't know what it did to the landing gear. So, I'm not going to retract it. We're going to fly in with the gear down. We're going to be going a lot slower than normal. I can only fly so fast with the gear extended."

He paused, reached up to the dash, and tapped a gauge. "I'm keeping an eye on the hydraulics. It's looking pretty good right now. But, like I said, I don't know what the strike did, if anything, to the landing gear. I've contacted dispatch and gave them an update. I've also contacted Sky Harbor tower to let them know the situation." Sky Harbor Airport is the name of the main international airport in Phoenix that we were going to.

"I've requested to do a fly by the tower to have them look at the landing gear to see what they can see," he went on. "I wanted you to know, so you're not wondering why we're flying past the airport."

I was not really sure how I felt right then. I was rather stunned that I didn't feel more nervous or concerned. Oddly, I didn't really feel any sense of dread or apprehension. I should have, but I didn't. I just nodded at what Shawn was telling me.

"Needless to say," Shawn continued, "make sure everything is securely fastened down back there. Just in case."

There was no panic apparent between these two up here. John had the protocol book open on his lap and was checking this and that. Shawn was focused and methodical in his actions. I felt reassured that everything was well handled.

"Let me know if you see or hear anything unusual back there en route," Shawn said before replacing his headset over his ear.

"Copy that," I said, as I did the same thing and turned around.

Chad was gazing at me with a quizzical look. Big boy was just snoring away with an occasional shift to get comfy, completely oblivious. I bent down on the way by Chad to tell him the news. He looked at me in disbelief.

"That's why I never heard the landing gear go up," he said. "I wondered if I just missed it."

Generally, you heard the gear retract and felt the thump as it closed. It was kind of a clue to us to know when it was okay to move around. I missed it too, but I just thought I wasn't paying attention. As a routine, we always kept everything secured in the back during flight, with the exception of my clipboard, our water bottles and maybe a book or something lying on a flat surface here or there. In the case of a violent transition, like a landing on the belly, any benign object, even a light one, can become a deadly missile flying through the cabin. Imagine what a simple water bottle could do to your head if it were to strike you. Ouch!

Chad and I flipped on the cabin lights and also got out the flashlights and started looking around at everything that was not securely fastened down or put away in a locking drawer.

Then we made sure our patient's restraining straps were tight.

The chart on this patient was uncomplicated and finished quickly, which gave me even more idle time to think about our landing. Amazingly, I wasn't feeling anxious at all. Thinking about our take off, I was surprised that I didn't feel the strike any more than I did. The landing gear on the Jetstream is anything but forgiving. They are hard and stiff. Again, thinking about landing in this aircraft, even the gentlest I've ever felt reminded me of slamming down on an aircraft carrier. It could possibly be smoother landing on the belly of the beast. There wasn't much else to do but sit and wait. Regardless of what was going to happen, there wasn't anything else I could do to change the situation. I was just going along for the ride. Chad was as calm as I was. We discussed it with shrugs of "whatever." To us at the time, it was more of an adventure than a concern.

The lights of Phoenix started to appear below us, indicating that it wouldn't be long now. Coming up on the airport, I heard the whine of the flap motors and felt the drag they produced. We dropped down to about 100 feet over the runway and passed by the tower out our left side. I checked on our sleeping giant, who shifted a little and made a snort without opening his eyes. He looked comfortable and his vital signs were clicking along unaltered. At the end of the airport, I felt the aircraft glide up a little in altitude and start to make a slow bank back around.

"Tower says the gear looks fine," Shawn said over the headset. His voice was smooth and subdued. Completely professional. "We're going to go on and give it a try. All secure in the back?"

"Copy that," I replied. "Slip this puppy up the runway, bro."

We had absolute confidence in Shawn's ability to bring us

in safely. Nevertheless, we still braced ourselves for touchdown. If this animal pounds the pavement with good landing gear, we could imagine its report with flawed gear.

All lined up on the final approach to the runway, the aircraft ever so slowly descended towards the asphalt. We were low and slow coming over the red leader lights before the numbers on the runway. I saw the numbers and painted chevrons slip underneath us. We were over the runway. We just seemed to be hanging there, mere feet before landing. Slowing, getting slower, hanging there, I was ready to feel what the landing gear did once we touched. Just slightly concerned now about the possible collapse of the struts and what that would do with our patient. How would the locking pins in the stretcher tolerate the kinetic energy of 380 pounds slamming across them?

Slowing even slower, just hanging there. I was waiting. Then, unexpectantly, the nose of the aircraft turned precisely into a taxi runoff. We were headed towards our parking tarmac. It wasn't until then that I realized that we were already on the ground. I literally never felt us touch or heard the bark of the tires. But we were on the ground headed to parking.

Once the pilot stopped getting instructions from ground control, I popped up on the intercom. "Whoa, dude, that was awesome!"

Chad followed it with, "Yeah, who's da man? Yup, that's right, you da man!"

We must have said it loud enough to wake up our happy camper. He looked over at us, utterly oblivious to the situation, with a big grin on his face after enjoying a delightful nap. Right about this time, I started to feel a mild *flump, flump, flump* coming from underneath us. We saw the ambulance to transport us to the hospital sitting by the gate as we pulled into our parking spot. Shawn glided the aircraft to a stop. More like it drifted up until it lost momentum. I didn't even feel that. After a couple of minutes to stabilize the engine pressures, I heard them rev up and shut off. Just like normal. As the propellers slowed down everyone went about their normal routine to offload a patient.

"You doing okay?" I asked our smiling friend.

"You bet," he spit out. "That was a great ride. You tell the pilot the drinks are on me." He started laughing. It made me wonder just how oblivious he really was. "Yeah, I felt like I was flying the whole way down here." He started laughing again.

Chad and I exchanged a humorous look at each other that, knowing each other as well as we did, said everything we felt that our patient didn't have a clue. Then Chad, in the voice of Fire Marshall Bill, commented on what we needed to do now that we were still alive, that had me unavoidably snickering. Grateful I hadn't just taken a drink of something, because it would be shooting out my nose.

It had John, who had gotten up and come back to open the door and set up the offload ramp, looking at us in wonderment. Right behind him was Shawn hurrying past to hop out the door. He didn't look at us, he was absorbed. You could hear the *beep, beep* of the ambulance backing up to the door, the cabin was aglow with the red brake lights as John fastened in the offload ramp for the stretcher. With a good bit of effort, Chad and I managed to budge our patient down to the ramp and slide him onto the ambulance gurney with assistance from John and the ambulance crew. On the way to the ambulance, I allowed the two burly EMTs to load the patient in the rig with Chad and John's assistance.

Unable to contain myself, I had to break away from the

loading of the patient to see what Shawn was looking at under the aircraft. Still not totally convinced that we actually did hit something coming off the ground. Maybe Shawn just thought he had. I wanted to know.

Shawn, with flashlight in hand, was staring at the nose gear. On the Jetstream, there are single tires on the main struts below the wings and the nose gear had two small tires in tandem attached to the single front strut. Both front tires were flat with a noticeable indentation of about two inches into the metal wheels. Oh yeah, we definitely hit something. We both exchanged glances in silence. Shaking my head, I turned to join the crew at the ambulance.

I passed John on the way to the ambulance. Nothing said, he had a huge smile on his face. Either from the joy of still being able to walk around right now, or from the amusement of our waggish patient. Rodney was entertaining, if anything. Everything ready to go, I hopped into the ambulance with everyone giggling and got ready for the ride to Phoenix Indian Medical Center. Now, after having a nap, our patient was rejuvenated and having a blast with all the attention. The ride into the hospital was uneventful but very loud with laughter. I believe we all got a little inebriated from the fumes emanating from the life of the party masquerading as a patient.

As much fun as we had with our large ball of cheery delight, the hospital staff didn't share our opinion. They did not seem amused at all. Which was rather depressing, leaving him there with them curtly telling him to settle down. Truth be told, all drunks are obnoxious. They can either be fun-loving obnoxious or they can be mean-spirited obnoxious. I prefer the former. He was definitely that. Chad and I told him goodbye and best of luck. As we walked away you could see that he was becoming more subdued, realizing the environment he was now relegated to was stern. If only we could tell them how much reason he had now to be this happy, but we couldn't.

We had a little piece of mind knowing that Rodney would probably do fine. Alcohol is one of those drugs that people build a tolerance to and this level was probably not that bad for him. He would be the patient you'd have to worry about if his ETOH level dropped below a certain level because he would go into withdrawals and delirium tremors, which could be even more dangerous.

By the time we got back to the airport Rick Heape was there along with a mechanic. They were all under the Jetstream assessing the damage. Chad and I put the empty flight stretcher back in the plane and joined them under the aircraft.

Rick looked at me with a wry smile, "Have a good flight back?"

"Yeah," I puckered, tilted my head a little and nodded. "Actually, I did."

"Did you know?" he asked.

"Yeah, Shawn told me right after we lifted. I wouldn't have known otherwise, though."

"Did you see the nose gear?" he asked Chad.

"No," Chad stepped up to look. "Dammmnnn! Guess we did hit something."

It turned out Shawn was right. An inspection of the gear showed the damage he was concerned about. Rick was livid —not at Shawn but at the transfer site. Someone on that team should have made certain the runway was safe and clear, and he wasted no time phoning the transfer site to demand just that in the future.

Watching that exchange, it dawned on me, this really could

have been bad. We got pretty lucky this time. Skinny ol' Chad walked up to Rick's six-foot three-inch bulk and draped an arm over his shoulder. He was looking at the mechanic working on the front wheels. He was standing there for a long moment, in silence, quietly nodding with his arm on Rick's shoulder. Eventually, Rick looked over at him wondering what the hell he was doing. Another second or two and Chad, with his lips tightly stretched over his teeth, looking remarkably like Jim Carrey in *The Mask*, stared up at Rick.

"So, Ricky," he said, sounding exactly how he looked. "Does this mean we're out of service for the night?"

"Why?" Rick looked at him amused. "You want to go home?"

"Uh, nope," Chad was shaking his head slightly exaggeratedly. "Nope. I want to go back to base and practice EMS." He stared up at him. "You know, Earn Money Sleeping."

"How do you propose we get there?" Rick said, allowing him to keep his arm on his shoulder.

Chad's facial expression dissolved. That took the wind out of his sail. But not to be disheartened, remaining in the same vocal characteristic, just softer now, "That do present a problem, now, don't it?" His arm slowly came off Rick's shoulder. "Umm, didn't think of that, now, did we?"

Rick walked off to talk to the mechanic, leaving Chad standing there.

"That was a damn good try, partner," I said to Chad, giving him a high-five. He shrugged.

A few minutes later Rick came back over. "Get in the van. I'll take you back to base. It's going to be a few hours to get this fixed at best. You're lucky, we have to go get parts."

I was sure Rick would have done it anyway, even if he didn't have to go get parts. It was just par for his character. Shawn and John stayed with the aircraft. The mechanic, Rob, hopped in the driver's seat of the company Suburban, Rick got in shotgun and Chad and I hopped in the backseats.

"What the hell happened up there?" Rick asked. I was sitting behind him and all I could see was the shine off the top of his hairless head. He was big enough to block about everything else out.

"I'm not sending any more of my people up there for anything until we know it's safe. I'm not risking my people for this silliness," Rick said.

His people, yup, his people. He didn't care about his airplane. No, it was about his people. It was easy to tell with Rick, it was about his people. I don't think he really had any concern right now about the business. To be honest, I think Rick was probably more shaken by this incident than any of the crew that was on the flight.

We got back to the hangar and Chad and I asked if they needed any help. Chad and I were there, we're on the clock, we didn't mind lending a hand if we could. But Rick and Rob had it in hand.

"No," Rick said, "you guys just go on and practice your EMS skills." Shaking his head at the thought of us sleeping while he was paying us. While he, the boss and owner of the whole company, was out driving around in the middle of the night fixing a wheel. "No. You guys go get yourself something to drink and go lay down. We got this. I need my crews to have their beauty sleep," he sarcastically said, walking to the maintenance hangar.

"Hey, will do, Ricky," Chad called out on the quiet, wide

open tarmac, watching for a reaction that he didn't get. "We'll just be in here. Let us know if you need any advice or anything. We got your back." Rick kept walking, but you could see his head drop and a little shake. There was the reaction Chad was going for, now he felt satiated.

In the morning, we came out and the Jetstream was sitting there all parked and hooked up on the auxiliaries. Looking like nothing ever happened last night. Shawn and John had already traded out their shift with the morning crew and were gone. So, we never had a chance, really, to praise them for a job well done. Even though we would have made it mordant and satirical. That's just our way. We'll catch them next time. Have no doubt.

Chapter 18
LAURA

While talking about the earlier years of this company, I would be remiss if I didn't mention Laura. When I first interviewed with NAAA, Laura was the Chief Flight Nurse. She was in charge of all the medical crews. A petite blonde girl, Laura was pretty. She was a relatively new nurse with ICU experience and very knowledgeable, mild-mannered, easy going. But more than that, she was classy. She was the epitome of an elegant, professional woman. She had a great deal of poise and presented an air of dignity. She was always in an agreeable demeanor, regardless of what was going on in her personal life. That was her character, and her character was supremely sophisticated. Even though she was young, she kept all her ducks in a row by keeping a fastidious eye on details. She was the ideal choice for a CFN, and I was always in awe of the fact that Rick had been able to obtain such an ideal person to take charge of his fledgling company.

Any other flight company would have hired her in a New York minute, but not as a manager. She had little managerial experience and no flight experience at the time she started with NAAA. In fact, she confided in me sometime later that she had purchased the book *Managing for Dummies*. She knew her limitations and knew how to overcome them. She was just the leader this company needed and every crew member respected her for that.

She insisted on doing a few shifts a month on the helicopter to keep her skills up, even though, she didn't have to. That was just the sort of team player she was. Besides, how better to know what the employees are going through than to be part of what they're going through yourself?

Being a young wife on top of being the Chief Flight Nurse, Laura did what many young wives do. She became pregnant. We didn't know it for a while. She let the cat out of the bag long before any of us would have picked up on it, though. To be honest, she never really showed until very late in her pregnancy. Even with her naturally thin body, she never really looked pregnant. Quite an achievement wearing a flightsuit!

She continued to fly almost until the day she delivered, regardless the toll it took on her. Every time she flew, she would get sick. Morning sickness and flying do not mix. Within minutes of taking off she would get sick and vomit. After which, she was perfectly fine and would continue the mission without flaw. Our barf bags became affectionately known as "Laura bags."

Before NAAA started up Native 5 at Deer Valley Airport in 1999, Chad had quit the company and moved to Kansas. Don't ask me why he went to Kansas. We kept in touch with that reasonably new and free medium of email. Occasionally, I'd still accept the expense of calling him, though. After one conversation, as we were closing, he told me to give Laura a pat on the butt for him.

The next day, I saw Laura walking across the tarmac in her

flightsuit with her medic partner. I knew that she loved Chad as much as I did and missed working with him as a partner. She was always wanting to know how he was doing. Not thinking about the consequences, I came up behind her and gave her a pat on the butt as directed.

"That was from Chad," I announced proudly. "He told me to do that the next time I see you."

She stopped, the look on her face was stunned disbelief. That wiped the smile off my face instantly. She was speechless and I was embarrassed. Trying desperately to dig myself out from under the bus, I said, "Chad told me to do that. It wasn't my idea. He said to tell you it came from him."

"But," she said, looking at me with scolding eyes, "it was your hand."

Shit, I was doomed. There was no way of turning back on this. What the hell was I thinking? "I'm sorry," I apologized, so profusely. "I was just doing what I was told."

"Well, that's a first," she countered sarcastically. "You tell Chad I'll deal with him later."

Dismissing it and me at the same time, she turned sharply and walked away. She maintained her position of authority. I couldn't be sure, though, but I think I might have detected just the slightest smirk on her face as she left. Regardless, she had put me in my place and I was going to have to tell Chad about it. When I did, he just laughed. He couldn't believe that I actually did it. Not to Laura. Was I crazy? Oh yeah, thanks a lot, *partner*!

When Laura was ready to step away from the demands of the CFN position and devote more time to her young family, she grabbed a spot on the line with the other flight nurses, away from managerial duties. It was my fortune that she stepped down when a nurse position opened at my base. I kind of think she planned it that way. There were two bases about the same distance from her residence. She picked Native 5. I think I know the reason, but I'm not telling, other than to say, it was the coolest base around, hands down. Being the CFN for the company since virtually the start, she knew the scoop on every base. There were no personality conflicts at our base, ever. No one heard much about us and we liked it that way. She fit in like a puzzle piece.

Laura had an impact on the base, for the better. She always had an impact on me. Her influence was to lead by example. She had an innate drive to always be better and to continue to advance in her career. Even with the full-time duty at work, she maintained a full-time duty as Mom at home. That notwithstanding, she also continued her own education. She maintained her position at Native 5 for a few more years before quitting and enrolling in a Nurse Practitioners program. She obtained that degree and continues until this day in that field. She continues to be an inspiration to everyone she meets. Just an example of what I tell people, the aeromedical field tends to attract some of the best of the best, but the best of the best are not all in the aeromedical field.

Chapter 19
THE LIFE, LOVE, AND RUMORS

Now, most of the people who worked within the very close-knit family of our aeromedical company were pretty restrained and monogamous. As I've said, there weren't many young people employed in this company. Most were married with families and were devoted to their off-duty families. Mostly. After all, the company was not staffed with machines. We were all human. And humans will be human regardless of their age and profession. When it came to innocent flirting, it was pretty common, even though it was "highly discouraged" by the front office. It was really obvious whose flirting was completely innocent and harmless, and whose was a little more questionable. It was also quite obvious who would take it well and who would not.

Medical personnel work in an environment that is awfully personal and very uncensored. It is our job to take care of the human body; all parts of the human body, specifically the naked human body. As discussed, it has become quite natural to ask a woman very personal questions like; how old are you, how much do you weight, and when was your last menstrual period? Not something anyone else would consider respectable queries of a perfect stranger. In this business, it's just par for the course. As a result, when you're being friendly with your peers, sometimes you get very close to the line of inappropriateness, however I was never short of people around me that would let me know when I was bumping the edge. I was really appreciative of that because I just didn't pay attention. It was not in my nature to think obscenely or offensively, but I love to play with the English language. As a result, my conversations would stumble into the risqué without knowing it.

While I was working down at the main base of the company at Williams Gateway Airfield, we had the fixed-wing crews sleeping quarters, all singular rooms, down one hall. But the rotor-wing crew shared a bedroom with a bunkbed. That was because they were dispatched with a hand-held radio at the time, before the Nextel phones. Not over the intercom in the main quarters. Also, their response needed to be more in sync, together and quick. So, it just worked out for us to be in the smaller room. So small that it demanded a bunkbed to be functional. None of us minded it. We all got along well together.

One day on coming in to work, it appeared that the top bunk was not used the previous night. The bottom bunk, however, seemed to have been used. When I left the day before, my partner and I had left the bunk sheets neat and tightly tucked. The top sheet was still as we left it, the bottom bunk was a mess. Though not ever actually spoken of, through clandestine glances and innuendos, it became apparent that not only was the bottom bunk used, it had been abused, frequently. Even though there was an earnest attempt to keep that information on the down low, it was well known within days throughout the company.

The singular use of only one of the bunkbeds didn't happen very often, at least to my knowledge. I'm sure it happened more often than I had knowledge of, though. I mean, given the environment we were in, the closeness, the nature of the work, and the opportunities, how could you be naïve to that? Occasionally, you'd hear things.

Rumor was that two of our flight nurses, a male and female, were having an affair. Working at one of our out-of-town bases, the female flight nurse thought she'd surprise the guy with a pleasant, unexpected visit. While he was out on a call, she decided to slip into his sleeping room and await his arrival. The gossip was that she was scantily clad; well, actually, she wasn't clad at all. Pure hearsay, mind you. She could hear as the helicopter was landing and was waiting for him in a rather provocative pose for him to enjoy coming into his room. Unbeknownst to her, when they returned, and him unaware of his present, he asked his male medic to get him something from his room. The medic not knowing that anyone else was in the quarters, walked into the room unannounced. Needless to say, he received the present that was *not* intended for him. What happened at a base, stayed at the base. At least, that was the way it was supposed to be. But this is the EMS industry and something like that just wasn't going to stay muted for long. Besides, it was funny.

In my own base, while I was still the manager, we had a flight nurse and a pilot become close. Both were single and unattached. But, again, everything was kept very discreet. In fact, these two were so inconspicuous that it wasn't until she was about six months pregnant that she finally decided to spill the beans. Knowing that she was going to become quite obvious shortly anyway. She let it be known that her and the pilot had been dating for some time now and were even living together. This came as a complete surprise to everyone at the base, who thought we knew everything about everybody there. Were we snookered! Well done, I commended her for his and her clandestine performance. Twelve years later, they're still unmarried, still living together, and are raising an extremely bright and well-adjusted son. Some combinations work well.

I was profoundly monogamous. As were all the other married personnel at my base. At least, if they weren't, it would have been an even bigger shock to me. Their wives were known and friendly with each other and would see each other at all the parties at Bud's house. So, if there was any fooling around on the side, I would have been amazed.

Well, except for one flight nurse at our base. He got a divorce, then got married, then got another divorce, then got married again. I'm sure there was probably some overlap in the process, but not to my personal knowledge. He seemed to just keep moving up until he latched onto one drop-dead-gorgeous, highly motivated, extremely intelligent girl a few years his junior. So, I can't really discredit him. He just wanted the best, he worked for the best, and he got the best. You go, boy!

Chapter 20
THE ANSWER IS *NO*

The EMS community is very close, especially flight crews, because we're just a smaller group, that's all. EMS deal with life situations that most people don't deal with. We get very close and personal about things that people don't get very close and personal about. We constantly deal with the full array of human emotions. We tend to see all angles and all perspectives that even we don't want to see sometimes. We discuss things that are generally kept completely with intimate friends.

As I was saying, our crews were relatively close, even the families. My wife came up to the base frequently to bring supplies she'd get for us at the store. As I was the base manager, it was my duty to supply the office materials and a few odds and ends, like cleaning supplies, that I'd get reimbursed for later by the company. Well, Susan would grab them and bring them up. All the guys knew her affectionately as the base mom.

One night after coming home from one of Bud's famous New Year's Eve parties, I was sitting on the back porch having a cigarette with Susan before retiring. We were talking about all the gossip we heard at the party. The wife of one of our pilots and Susan were particularly close this night and spent most of the night talking together. Knowing that Susan was considered the base mom, she thought that Susan might have some insight into the people at the base.

In the midst of our conversation, Susan said, "She asked me if I thought her husband would ever fool around on her." Girl talk, you know. She paused while she took a sip. "I told her, no. He just didn't seem to be the type." She looked at me for confirmation. "Do you think he would?"

"No," I replied succinctly. "He definitely notices good-looking women. He may think about it. Though he's never indicated it to me. Hey, we're guys. Like I've always said, you don't stop window shopping when your married. If he stops looking at women, she's the one that'll suffer. It either means he's no longer interested in sex. Or he's no longer interested in sex with women."

That seemed to pacify her. She flipped her cigarette on the ashtray, and not looking up, she casually asked, "Would you ever fool around on me?"

Remember, I've just finished coming home from a great New Year's Eve party.

"Well," I started, "if I was in Seattle, Washington, a long way from home. By myself, in a hotel room where no one else could possibly see the door. Late at night. And I hear a knock on the door and it's Salma Hayek, butt naked, and she says, 'Don't say anything. I just want to have sex.' Would I break down and give in? Yeah, probably. But the chances of that happening are one in never in this universe."

Feeling like I explained myself pretty well, I looked up at her and she was looking at me. If you've ever been married, you know the look I was getting right then. Gentlemen, in case you don't know it, the answer to the question your wife asks you about fooling around on her is: No. Don't try to negotiate it, don't try to manipulate it, don't try to justify it. It's simple. No, of course not. "No, honey, never." The answer is simply *No*.

It wouldn't be the first time my blatant honesty had gotten me in trouble and I was sure it would not be the last time either. I have no filter between my brain and my mouth. If I'm thinking it, it just comes out. But even when you're a little tipsy, gentlemen, use some discretion. It's better for everyone in the long-run. Fucking mouth.

Regardless of what happened the day before, the night before, or even the morning of, when I'd leave for work everything was settled. That was the one thing I can say about Susan and me. We never let loose ends ride when I went to work. Because, both of us knew it was always possible that I may not come back home. We always kissed and said, "I love you," before I jumped in the car for work. That was the one thing that was a little unique about working in the aeromedical environment, you thought about things like that. Anybody could go to work and not come back. In any profession. But we did think about it. That was different.

Chapter 21
DON'T TELL ANYONE

I really shouldn't be telling you this because what happens in the aircraft with flight crews should stay in the aircraft with flight crews. It's a very veiled world for a reason. We deal with life and death. We deal with the unsightly and darker side of life. We deal with the extremes of emotions, of others and ourselves. It is the nature of the business. Not so very different from other emergency services like firefighters, paramedics, and law enforcement personnel. But there are things that we do to keep our sanity. Often, it is just silly little pranks we play on our follow colleagues that attempt to introduce fun into what can be a very chaotic and disturbing world.

In the early days of NAAA, we didn't have a myriad of rules and regulations within the company. We were a small bunch of folks all working to make a viable, efficient, elevated company in the aeromedical field. We wanted to be the best and bring the best in a very demanding and scrutinized industry. At that time, we didn't have a lot of company regulations because we didn't need them. The company didn't need to tell the employees to act professionally, we did that on our own. If someone didn't, the other crews would confront him or her personally. What everyone did reflected directly on everyone else. The company didn't feel the need to tell us to continue our education and obtain certifications that would make us better, we did that on our own. The personnel that NAAA obtained, after starting the rotor program were some of the best. Some came from other flight companies or were very long-time experienced nurses and medics that wanted to get into flight.

Some of the first crews had military backgrounds. One of our nurses was a Navy Seal, one was from the Army Special Forces, a Green Beret, one of our medics was a sniper in the Army. I was from the Army Airborne. Some of our nurses were well advanced in their career. One of our nurses was a certified mid-wife.

Now, the helicopter pilots were another highly-skilled bunch as well. All handpicked by the very demanding and fastidious Chief Helicopter Pilot and director of the rotor program, Coffey. He knew most of the helicopter pilots in the valley and picked the very best to work with this new startup company. He knew the best, he wanted the best and he got the best. All of them had tons of flight time, mostly from other aeromedical companies or from news channel helicopters.

Because of this, when we did our job, we were focused and meticulous. All of us. We didn't have to be told. But when we were not involved in a medical mission, we had fun. There are a few ways to have fun, especially when you have a helicopter at your disposal and the entire state of Arizona below you.

On occasion, we'd land on the top of a high mesa where you can get a great view, the top would be less than a quarter of an acre in area. Then, if the pilot was really feeling frisky, when you lifted off the mesa, he'd keep the helicopter just a few feet off the ground until you cleared the edge of the mesa and it dropped away precipitously. Then he'd suddenly drop the nose down to obtain speed and all of your senses would start screaming.

One time, we were taking a patient to the VA hospital in Prescott and coming back empty. Knowing this before we left, we bagged up a couple of sandwiches. On the way home, we landed on the top of a plateau just north of Black Canyon City, where the pilot knew of some old Native American ruins. We sat there and had lunch in a place that you could only get to after a full day's hike. Unless you had a helicopter.

Sporadically, when we were returning to base and coming over a fellow crew members house, that was off for the night, the pilot would gradually decrease altitude to about three hundred feet until he was directly over their residence and then pull pitch, increasing the angle of the rotor blades that produced upward thrust and pull up at the same time. That would create a tremendous *thump, thump, thump* and that would almost rattle the windows below. We wouldn't do it in the wee hours of the morning, of course, because of the neighbors. But our fellow flight crew members would know when their colleagues were overhead.

Our pilots were always cautious, with a mind on safety, but there were things that you could do with a helicopter that pilots wouldn't do with patients or the general public on board. That being said, all the pilots knew all the medical crews and what they were willing to do and their comfort levels. They would never make abrupt maneuvers, even if only one of the crew was uncomfortable with it. They could be extremely gentle when gliding the aircraft through the sky. Weather permitting.

To let the pilot know that the medical crew was cool with having a little fun, I would say something to the effect of,

"Everything is well secured back here. In case you have to make any abrupt maneuvers. Just so you know." They'd understand the implication.

With the right crew, a call cancelled en route and a return to base could produce rather fun results. If we were out over the open desert, the pilot might pull the aircraft sharply into a vertical ascent, pointing straight up into the air. Shooting up like an arrow. Just as the aircraft lost forward momentum, he'd push the tail rotor hard, making the nose swing around, pointing straight down. Pointed directly at the ground, the aircraft would fall, rapidly gaining speed until you were at the altitude you wanted then he'd pull the nose back up and you were magically headed right back where you came from. This was known as a "hammerhead" maneuver. Better than any rollercoaster rides you've ever been on because this puppy wasn't attached to rails. The sensation was exhilarating. It had the power to make grown men scream in delight like a couple of pre-adolescent girls. Or they could take the more traditional route and just bank around to return to base, but not that gentle, wide bank that the general public would get. Oh, no. It would be a hard-ninety-degree bank where you're looking out the left window straight at the ground and the right window was straight up into the air. You were completely sideways. The impressive thing about that was, no matter how sharp the turn was, if a spare IV bag was hanging from the ceiling it would not swing. It always hung straight down to the floor. Regardless of the orientation of the floor, parallel or perpendicular with the earth. It didn't pull to one side or the other, it was always straight down. Because the G forces were straight down. I never felt sick in a helicopter. Ever. No matter what we did. There were times when I'd be in the fixed-wing airplane that I would get a little queasy.

The fixed-wing side of the company would have their fun also, of course, depending on the pilot and crew. When we first started, we had the Jetstream aircraft. It was a large, for aeromedical anyway, aircraft and was built sturdy. Its original design was to ferry British military personnel out to aircraft carriers. Hence the frame and landing gear were a little more beefy than usual. It also required two pilots, a captain and first officer, at all times. Because of the design, the aircraft could tolerate more in maneuvers than other airplanes. With the right crew, it wasn't unusual to be flying along, without a patient on board and have the pilot put the plane into zero Gs by descending at a particularly steep rate. It was an absolute blast to float through the cabin completely weightless. But, at the bottom of the arc, they'd have to pull up relatively hard increasing the G force considerably. That, on occasion would make me a little queasy. Not enough to ever make me decline to agree to the maneuver though. The only other time I might get just a little unsettled would be in heavy weather, where the aircraft would be riding up and down on the wind and air pockets. Helicopters didn't do that much. They stayed relatively steady in most weather. At least that was the way it felt. That was because, as the pilots put it, airplanes ride on the whims of the wind and helicopters beat the wind into submission. Turbulence didn't affect helicopters as dramatically as it did airplanes.

One day, on the way up to San Carlos Indian Reservation for a call, I was riding with our finest pilot and Mike Q. as the medic. Flying along, strictly by the book, heading to San Carlos directly, point A to point B. I was preparing my chart in a relaxed manner knowing I had plenty of time. The pilot switched on a country-western station on one of the bands on the radio and we listened to the static-filled music to kill time. These radios were not built nor were they very good at picking up music radio stations, but it was something. About twenty miles out of San Carlos, dispatch notified us that we were cancelled. The patient had declined to be transferred to a hospital in Phoenix. Despite the doctor's suggestion, the patient flatly refused to be transferred to another hospital. So, we turned around.

As we were heading back to base, I remembered hearing a little gossip from another crew about flying through Rogers Canyon. I knew Mike was of an adventurous nature and so was I, so just in passing, I sort of made mention that Rogers Canyon was on the way home. Wasn't it? The pilot realized immediately what I was alluding to.

"Do you want to go through the canyon, Cletus?" he asked me, knowing exactly what I wanted.

"Uh," I hesitantly responded, trying not to sound excited, "Sure."

I looked at Mike, whose eyes were wide with a big shit-eating smile below them. I'm sure it was a mirror of my own face.

"Well, make sure your seatbelts are tight. It's coming up."

Mike and I grabbed our seatbelts and cinched them tight, then suddenly, we dropped down. We dipped below the rim of the canyon and well into it, reminding me of the scene from *Star Wars* going down in the canyon of the Death Star. But this canyon wasn't straight. It turned sharply from side to side, and we followed it turn for turn with hard banks to stay in the center. My right hand shot up to the ceiling and my left grabbed Mike's shoulder to brace myself instinctively. In fact, I didn't need to. Even with the hard, quick banking, the G-force was always pushing down to the floor. In reality, I could have just sat there literally drinking a cup of coffee and never spilled a drop. But the visual effect was so awesome that this beat any thrill ride I'd ever been on. I was screaming and laughing so hard at the same time that before long it was hard to catch my breath. I started screeching, "I need oxygen. I need oxygen." In between my gasps of utter exhilaration. This pilot was a pro at making Little Girl perform at her best, like she was an extension of his own body. The two were so in sync with each other that it gave you total confidence, all the while you're shrieking in delightful terror. I was laughing so hard my abdomen started to cramp up. In fact, it was contracted so hard it pushed my diaphragm up to the point I couldn't inhale. But with the intense abdominal pressure and nowhere for the air in my gut to go, I started farting. I was laughing so hard, I was farting. Which only increased the humor and brought hilarious comments from the pilot. The only one of us that was experienced enough with this that he could still talk normally.

We didn't stay down in the canyon for very long, only a few miles, just a minute or two, but it was without a doubt the most thrilling moment of my life. Thank the universe and all the wonders that be, because I couldn't have gone much longer without catching my breath. Was I ever concerned for my safety? No, never. Not once. Were we all taking a chance? Yes, absolutely. Would anyone in the office ever condone such actions? Are you kidding? If anyone ever found out about this, it would have been condemned as a frivolous and completely dangerous action. Highly frowned upon by any governing authorities. But it was like being in the stunt in an action movie. It was something that most people would never get to do and with a pilot who I had complete and utter faith in with my life. It was, in a word, a *trip*. Would it have scared the shit out of most people? Yup. But for us, it was incredibly fun. It was what made this job so pleasurable. You can't get away with that kind of fun these days. The helicopters have GPS tracking devices on them and the flight track can be seen. But that day was one of the best. It took me the rest of the way back to base to recover my breathing. My abdomen and face were sore the whole next day. And, I wouldn't have traded that day for a year's paycheck. That was what made working here, with these crews, the best time of my life.

Just don't tell anyone.

Chapter 22
OH, CRIKEY

That night, after the day flying through the canyon, Fred, the night pilot, came on and took the night shift. Pilots can only work twelve-hour shifts. So, we'd work with two pilots during our twenty-four-hour shift. Fred was an interesting individual. Very laid back, older guy getting close to retirement like Bud. He was a pretty good size boy. One not to be worried about the pounds when there was something good to eat. However, looking at him, you would never consider him obese or out of shape. He carried it very well and looked fit. I rarely ever saw him without his smoking pipe stuffed under a full salt-and-pepper mustache.

Standing protocol was that you didn't drink eight hours before your shift and no smoking within fifty feet of the aircraft. We always jokingly expressed it backward with, no smoking within eight hours of your shift and no drinking within fifty feet of the aircraft. When we were put on standby, our normal Standard Operating Procedure was to go to the aircraft and wait by it until scrambled. I always use to stand at least fifty feet away and have a cigarette before launching. Fred would lean up against the nose of the aircraft and smoke his pipe. I asked him about that one time and he replied, "Oh, yeah, that 1,800-degree exhaust coming out of that tail pipe is not going to ignite the fuel and oxygen tank in the aircraft that's sitting right under it, but me up here at the nose, smoking my 300-degree pipe might just blow us up." Then he'd give me that look. That was the only regulation or protocol, Fred would skirt. I had been told before that I could probably light my cigarette off the exhaust pipe, but I never tried.

Fred had been around awhile. He joined the Army the year I was born. Word was that he was the first helicopter pilot in the Vietnam War to be awarded the Medal of Honor. When you'd ask him about it, he was very quiet. When you'd ask him how he got it, he was always aloof. "I just did my job," was about the most you'd ever get him to say about it. I finally had to look on the Internet to find the story he would never disclose. It just didn't seem to be something he wanted to talk about, and I respected that and didn't push. He was a reserve, very humble guy. Didn't joke around. Didn't play around. When he flew, it was from point A to point B by the book, following regulations. He never wavered. He was always very pleasant, a man who enjoyed the little things in life, but he pretty much kept to himself. He didn't do "fun things" like some of the other pilots. For him it was strictly business, and you always knew it was going to be strictly business, so don't ask.

Tonight, a little late in the evening, we were put on standby for an MVA down south on Interstate 10. We all gathered at the aircraft, and I no sooner lit up a cigarette when the radio blurted out to scramble. That was quick, no fooling around here. Within seconds, we were onboard, secured and off the ground. Fred, true to form, cleared our departure with the airport tower and took off in textbook fashion, radioed dispatch our departure, and received further instructions to the scene.

The fire department had all of the right-side lanes of this four-lane stretch blocked off at the accident site, backing up traffic for miles. Arizona State Troopers were directing traffic down just one lane on the far-left side of the Interstate. There were three cars involved in the smash up, one in the first lane still attached to another at the bumpers in the emergency lane and one a short distance away, off the road going up an embankment. We landed just south of the mayhem. Walking up, I glanced at the vehicles to get an idea of the mechanisms involved in this accident, trying to figure out who hit who and what kind of impact force was sustained. There was a pick-up truck with an SUV with not much rear end left on it crammed into the truck's bed. On the hill was what looked like a relatively compressed black Mustang. As I came up on the scene where all the white lights had been directed into, the incident commander guided us to our patient.

This is not one of those times when I was going to casually get a report from the paramedic while my partner assessed the patient. This time, we were going straight to all hands-on board, *lifesaving skills in progress*. There were several paramedics and firefighters that were rendering aid to an older gentleman, about fifty years old, who was laid on his back. One was putting in an IV, another was holding a mask down on his face while another was using an ambu bag to breathe for this guy. One was holding pressure on his bleeding leg while another was wrapping a trauma dressing over the wound. This guy was a mess.

In EMS, there are really only two kinds of calls; "Oh, shit" calls and "Bullshit" calls. When you first walk up on a scene, your experience tends to give you a feeling of either, "Yeah, this is busy but we'll be okay," or, "Oh, shit!" This was of the "Oh, shit" variety. This was where I let my training and experience take over.

First thing you want to do coming up to your patient is a primary survey, which, essentially, is to establish if the patient is awake, has a patent airway, is breathing, and has a heartbeat. As I knelt down by the paramedic bagging the guy, everything was answered in a second. He was not awake, there was blood blowing up into the mask with every squeeze on the bag and a quick glance at the monitor showed he had a steady heartbeat. The blood in the mask was my first and primary concern. Every few breaths they bagged into the man, the responder holding the mask would lift it, and, using the portable suction they very smartly brought to the scene, cleared his airway of the incessant blood. Where was all the blood coming from?

"What have we got here?" I asked.

"Unrestrained driver of that Cadillac," the paramedic informed me. "Positive LOC, we removed him from the vehicle and hooked him up on the monitor. Multiple cuts to the face. He's trying to breathe, but he has an obstruction in his mouth."

Wait a minute, what Cadillac? Was that crumpled up Mustang really a full-size Cadillac? Just a brief passing thought.

I grabbed the intubation kit and started preparing to insert a breathing tube into this guy. With that amount of blood coming out of the mouth, this man needed a definitive airway just so he wouldn't aspirate all of this blood into his lungs. I didn't want him filling his lungs with blood from wherever it was coming from with every inhalation.

"Good luck with that," the paramedic commented.

That's never a good sign when they say something like that.

They were doing a pretty good job keeping the man's oxygen saturation up, but this just wasn't going to last. Especially not through the flight to the trauma center. When I was ready and Mike was standing by to assist, I got into position.

"Okay," I said, "let's take a look. Have the suction ready."

Just as I put the laryngoscope into his mouth, I could see the reason for all the blood. It made my heart skip a beat, or maybe even two. Lodged in the base of his throat was a chunk of glass, possibly part of the windshield. Wherever it came from, it was not coming out without causing catastrophic damage. This was not a good thing. I removed the laryngoscope blade, suctioned his mouth clear, and had them continue on with what they were doing.

"We're going to have to cric this guy," I said, looking at Mike. Without flinching, Mike reached for the trauma bag to pull out the cric kit.

Doing a cricothyroidotomy, or a cric for short, is cutting a hole directly into the throat in the front just under the Adam's apple. It is a lifesaving procedure that is never considered lightly for obvious reasons. I have been trained to do this procedure since I was a medic in the Army. Over and over, trained and practiced on many a cadaver, pig parts, and mannequins. Over thirty years of training to do this one procedure. But, up to this point, I have never had to do it. Even though I was all calm and cool on the outside, you can just imagine where my underwear was at this point.

While Mike was getting the cric kit pulled out, I reached down into my calf pocket and pulled out my narcotics bag. I tossed a vial of morphine and a sedative with syringes to the medic manning the IV. I noted on the monitor that this man was maintaining a respectable blood pressure despite blood from the mouth, the face, the leg, and God knows where else in his body. I asked the medic to draw up a certain amount of narcotic and sedative, a light dose, and give it. I trusted the scene paramedics and they never let me down to do just what I asked. Even though the patient was unresponsive at this time, I didn't want him waking up from the pain of me cutting his throat open. That would be a bad time to start coming around.

I positioned myself in the most optimum position to perform this procedure as I'd practiced all of my career. I put my fingers on his throat and identified my landmarks on his neck that showed me where to make my incision, took the scalpel, along with a deep breath, and made the cut. I was pleasantly surprised to have minimal bleeding. Certainly, not as much as was coming from the mouth. I took the scalpel and punctured the membrane I needed to get through. A *bougie* is a long, soft, malleable plastic covered wire about half the thickness of a pencil. I stuck a bougie in the hole I just made so I wouldn't lose the entrance to the trachea, I held up my hand and Mike placed the intubation tube in it like a trained scrub nurse. I slid the intubation tube over the bougie and pushed it in through the opening in the neck, putting it in just far enough to inflate the securing balloon. The paramedic bagging the patient switched the bag from the mask to the tube now. Mike, with stethoscope already in his ears, listened to confirm I had good breath sounds in both lungs of the patient. Now, I could breathe again. The procedure went along just as I'd been taught and practiced. What a relief! Now, let's get this guy secured and out of here to the trauma center.

Wasting no time, I fastened the cric tube securely to the man's neck with pleading instructions to everyone not to let the thing come out. While that was going on, another large bore IV was inserted with another bag of fluids going. Other firefighters made sure the guy was secured to the backboard. Within minutes we were off to the waiting aircraft with four stout firefighters on each corner of the backboard, Mike holding the tube to make sure it didn't move, and the paramedic bagging breaths into the guy with another firefighter following, carrying the oxygen tank and monitor. Me, I was following behind watching everything like an apprehensive mother. I didn't want one little slip, or one IV or oxygen tube, getting caught someplace it shouldn't be, to accidently cause anything to get pulled out. Especially, the cric tube.

The incident commander walked up to me as we were going by and handed me a sheet of paper. "This is all the information I got on the guy," he said. "Name and date of birth is about all I could get."

"Great," I told him in earnest. "I'm happy to get that. How'd you get it?"

"Driver's license." Then, he held out a wallet. "Here, you might as well take this."

I thanked him again as he followed me up to the aircraft. Just before we came under the rotor disk, feeling pretty confident that everything was in order and not going to get pulled, I darted around to open the door and get ready to load. When the top rotors are spinning around they look like a disk, and once underneath, it's difficult to communicate verbally. We loaded the patient without incident and I thanked everyone for their good work. Everything secured, I climbed in.

"Let me know when we're good to go," Fred said over the intercom.

I took over bagging while Mike got strapped in, then he took over while I strapped in.

"Good to go," I announced. "Forty-five-year-old, male, 220 pounds, going to Maricopa County with a cold off-load. We'll patch en route. But we're good. Hit it."

Fred gently coaxed Little Girl into the air and off we went. I pulled out the AutoVent and set it up. The AutoVent is a small, very basic ventilator that could take over the ventilations for the patient and free up Mike's hands for other things. Although, truth be told, there wasn't really much else to do for this man. His vital signs were all looking pretty good on the monitor, IVs were dripping, and the bleeding was getting controlled with Mike suctioning the mouth only occasionally. Now, that it wasn't being hammered by the ambu-bag through his mouth to keep him breathing, the bleeding had slowed some. Both of us applied dressings to the multiple face and head lacerations. I patched into Maricopa County Medical Center over the radio and let them know what was coming and when we'd be there. Minutes later we landed.

Some pilots would think this stuff was pretty cool and come into the trauma bay with us to watch. Not Fred. He had no interest, he'd been there, done that. He stayed out by the aircraft and smoked his pipe while he waited.

Once in the trauma bay, I called out the report. "Any questions?"

"Why'd you cric him?" the doctor asked.

"Airway obstruction," I responded. I had given in report that there was glass in the mouth. Sometimes, with as busy as it gets in the trauma room, some information gets missed; sometimes it just doesn't register. The glass chuck in his mouth had completely obstructed his airway.

"What obstruction?" the doctor questioned.

"I think it's a piece of windshield. Not sure. But there's a chunk of glass in the back of his throat."

"Oh yeah, you did say that." The doctor nodded, remembering. "Well, that should make things interesting. Any idea how the glass got down his throat?"

I wanted so much to say something like, 'Well, doc, I guess when his head slammed through the windshield, he probably thought he'd just bite off a chunk of glass to see how it tasted.' I wanted to, but of course I didn't. I just looked at him and shrugged. I knew the question was rhetorical.

"I think that'll get it. Thanks. Strong work," he said.

I had the recording nurse sign my unfinished chart and timed it. "Let me go write this and I'll bring you back a copy," I told her. She nodded absently, keeping her eyes focused on what the trauma team was doing and writing that down.

"Now for the fun part," I said to myself sarcastically. From the time we got the call, to the time we flew to the scene, to the time on the scene with all the procedures we did, to the time it took to fly to the trauma center, up to now was forty-seven minutes. I was easily going to spend the next sixty minutes trying to chart everything accurately. On this one, you had to make sure everything that was done is in order, all the I's dotted, all the T's crossed, all the reasons explained and all the procedures and treatments precisely documented in detail. This chart was sure to be scrutinized and mulled over and picked apart for any discrepancies. It ended up taking me over eighty minutes to write the chart. Almost twice as long as the actual call. I took pride on the fact that it didn't take me long to write charts, normally, but this one was special. Somewhat unusual and certainly involved. It was nowhere near routine, so I had to stop and think about certain aspects that had to be charted.

I found Mike in the EMS room and we walked out together.

Fred was outside the helipad fence, puffing on his pipe. While I was charting, Mike had come out and cleaned and readied the aircraft.

"Well," I commented as usual, "that's a save."

"That was a bloody mess," Mike stewed. "I just got it all cleaned up before you came out. Not bad, though, first actual cric I've seen done in the field."

I turned to Mike when we got to the gate, "Hey, that paramedic said that guy was in the Cadillac. I thought the black car was a Mustang or Altima or something. Didn't look like a full-sized Cadillac."

"Yeah, it was pretty squashed," Mike agreed. "Might have been a Cadillac, but it's pretty compact now."

On the way back to base, Mike and I engaged in different conversations. A little about the call, a little about other flight crew members. Fred remained silent except for necessary transmissions on the radio. All I could see of him was his silhouette backlit from the instrument panel. The unlit pipe sticking out of the side of his mouth.

Somehow, Mike and I got on the subject of pilots. Not even considering that Fred could hear everything we said. Forgot he was there in his silence. I was telling Mike how safe I felt with the pilots Coffey had at this company. And not just because they're all really good pilots, but because none of them were suicidal. I was jesting that as long as they weren't suicidal, they wanted to get their own butt back home safely. In the process, they're going to get my butt back safely too. They may not be trying consciously to save my life, but they are definitely consciously trying to save their lives. Mike was nodding agreement and stating as much also.

About an eight-mile radius around Williams Gateway

Airport was a non-populated area with cow pastures and cotton fields. There was a good stretch getting close to the airport that is blacker than the pit to hell below us and it was hard to make out just how high off the ground we were. It was quiet for a minute as I looked out into the unknown darkness.

Unexpectedly, Fred, in a solemn voice, came over the intercom. "Hey, Kurt, did I tell you that my wife was leaving me?"

Stunned, I answered, "No. You didn't." I was caught off-guard. Saddened. I didn't know if I should inquire as to why or just let it be. It felt a little personal to ask, especially with Fred being a private sort of guy.

"Yeah," he continued, "she said she didn't want to put up with me now that she knows I have stage four cancer in the brain."

Abruptly, the nose of the aircraft was pointed straight down and precipitously dove into the black abyss below us. With that bodily instinct of my arms flying out to grab something as we plummeted to our death, all you could hear in the aircraft was Mike and me yelling, "Aaaahhhh!" It was loud and the intercom was off. We could be heard past the earpiece covering the headset.

It was so completely out of character for Fred. Or maybe completely in character for Fred and we just never knew it. Slowly the helicopter leveled out and regained altitude.

A subdued voice came back over the intercom with, "Just kidding."

I looked up at the silhouette of Fred with the pipe shape moving up and out a little bit indicating a tremendous grin growing on his face.

"Good one, Fred," I laughed out.

"Yeah, good one," Mike added. "But now I'm going to have to spend another hour cleaning up the inside … again."

Fred remained quiet the rest of the way into base while Mike and I couldn't stop laughing. Oh yeah, that was a good one. Got us there. That's why I love this job. Fucking pilots.

Chapter 23
RICK HEAPE

Rick had started Native American Air Ambulance after the situation at his current employment changed. He was employed as a captain for America West Airlines and was invested with retirement and stock options when the company was sold, changing the whole dynamics of the employees' retirement and pension funding. Taking a huge risk, he invested all his money, along with some family funds, in to start a new aeromedical company. An aeromedical company is a reasonably complex endeavor. There's a lot of aspects that go along with a medical aviation company. Not just all the parts and pieces, but the licenses and permits that go along with each one. Aviation and medical are both rife with regulations, local, state, and federal. Not to mention, he was starting an aeromedical company in the middle of two other aeromedical companies' area and the field is highly competitive. It was not an easy enterprise. But he was able to do it. In fact, he did it so well that within five years, he owned the largest aeromedical company in Arizona. He even surpassed an established company that had been here for over twenty-five years. He was magnanimous to admit that it wasn't his ingenuity and brilliance only that achieved this feat. He gave the majority of the credit to the people working for him. Or, as he put it, working with him.

He had a few along the way that didn't do him any service, who tried to run the company like a high-priced, money-grubbing corporation. A couple of people who had positions of authority who wanted to strongarm the employees to push harder and make less money. They wanted them to take on extra roles, do extra work all in the name of the good of the company. I daresay, it was not what they would have asked of themselves. But it made them look good on the bottom line. As soon as Rick found out what was going on, he stepped in. In most cases, the offending authority figure was let go. Occasionally, they were just demoted and put back into the pool of the other employees. Rick had a philosophy of how he wanted his company ran and he wasn't going to let net profits supersede his vision.

We were talking one night outside in the cool March air and I mentioned to him in all honesty. "You know, if you wanted to, you could easily make a seven-figure salary from this company."

"Yeah," he responded, "I probably could. But that's not what I'm about. I just want it to succeed beyond my wildest dreams." He paused for a moment of contemplation. "And, so far, it has." A proud smile crossed his face. It seemed Rick didn't measure success in personal financial gains but rather in the good he could do and the accomplishments he could make. He was making the lives of other people better and he took pride in that. His company was providing a better service than the competition and that gave him the satisfaction of success.

At that time, Rick was still working full-time at his normal flight company as a senior captain. He was only doing NAAA part-time, even though he was here almost all of the time. It was a few years before he finally quit his other position and devoted himself full-time to NAAA. That's when the company really started to grow rapidly. He got rid of the Jetstream airplanes and replaced them with the Pilatus PC-12, one of the first companies in the United States to utilize them for aeromedical. The Pilatus PC-12 is an aeromedical dream bird, it's extremely cost-effective and flies like a homesick angel. The aircraft had incredible capabilities for being a single-engine aircraft. It had a fantastic climb rate, long-range capacity, and maneuvering abilities. Plenty of room inside for patient care and a huge cargo door that made loading a patient a breeze. It was fast too. This single turbo-prop aircraft looked like a Mako shark. It had a trailing link landing gear, which meant when it touched down, it felt like it was on a cushion. Sweet! Rick even started to put up his own helicopter bases, apart from Omniflight, completely owned and operated by NAAA. He was going strong, for a while, at least.

Because of the events that happened in Rick's life, namely home life involving a divorce, it became time for him to relinquish and sell off Native Air in order to divide his assets. It was what was best for him at this juncture. He sold the company to Omniflight Helicopters, the company that was already partnered with him supplying the helicopter component of the business. Now they just acquired the whole thing. It was the end of an era. A cherished era that I would never see again.

When Omniflight took over, the whole environment changed. Now it wasn't a company owned and operated by one man, it was a corporation. It was no longer a family. It was big business, complete with a hierarchy of people in charge, who didn't even live in the state. Investors were where the monetary buck really stopped. Only with a corporation, the responsibility buck really never stops. It just keeps getting passed along. The beauty with Rick was when there was a problem, you knew who to go to. You knew where the end of the line was. He couldn't pass anything off as, "They won't let me." If something needed to be done or changed, Rick had the power to do it. Without exception and without a committee. That made working for him enjoyable. Because of that, and because of the way Rick was, every crew member felt a vested interest in this company. We all had a feeling of a certain individual pride and took figurative ownership of the operation of Native Air. As Rick would always say, "This is your company, make it the best." We did. When the crews talked about the company, it was always in the context of "my company." Now it belonged to someone else. And it became quite obvious very quickly that the only person this new corporation was interested in was George Washington.

I asked Rick one time how he built such a great company in such a short time. He thought about it for a while, then answered, "I think it was divine intervention. Really, I don't know how I got so lucky. All the pieces just seemed to fall in the right place at the right time. I really do think it was inspired." I had to agree with him, it was miraculous.

Even the medical director he was able to obtain was an inspirational gift. Dr. Shufeldt was the proverbial overachiever, an emergency room doctor with a law degree and, on top of everything else, an avid pilot with his own plane. He immersed himself in the duties of medical director for the company in all aspects, from protocols to the education of the teams and was always available to every employee. To this day, even as busy as he is constantly, if I call him on the phone I rarely get voicemail; *he* answers.

Rick said once, *"It's amazing what you can accomplish when you don't care who gets the credit."* Rick was gracious and grateful, but that didn't stop him from enjoying the benefits he had reaped from his hard work. He enjoyed the perks that being the owner of a company like this afforded him while he owned it. After he sold it, he took his proceeds and started living the life he wanted to. He had himself a beautiful new girlfriend, he was negotiating the purchase of a new yacht, and he was starting a new business adventure. Yup, he was living the life.

I didn't hold any animosity toward him for selling. I had seen this guy help everyone in the company in everyway he could. I have seen him give loans or advances, if you will, to employees who were struggling through hard times. Many of which would soon after quit the company without paying back his generosity. I heard him say, "Never again. I'll never do that again." Only to do it again. And again, and again. That was just his nature. But now he was able to put all that aside and live for himself. Good for you. You go, boy!

Two years later, I was hit with the news that Rick had suffered a major heart attack while vacationing in Sedona. I was struck dumbfounded when I learned he hadn't survived it, the news was unbelievable. He'd finally weathered the development of a successful flight company, with all of its mysterious peaks and valleys, and now this. He wasn't old, either. In fact, he was in the prime of his life. I was deeply saddened about the news because of the feelings it generated in me. For a boss, an employer, an owner of a company, a man driven to be successful, even with all the faults of any human, Rick was a good man. I have never had a boss like him before in my career and haven't since. He was unique. Someone I considered a good friend. His passing was untimely and unexpected. It created an emptiness in my heart and really seemed the final curtain to the former and beloved Native American Air Ambulance that I knew. I will miss him, all the memories with him and everything he represented.

Chapter 24
CHANGE

The only thing that doesn't change in the aeromedical profession is continuous change. Being on the forefront of advanced research, rapid improvements with new drugs, new equipment and new procedures was a consistent way of life. Things change so fast that it was a challenge to just keep up. That's why everyone in the aeromedical profession is in a steady state of education, training, reeducation, and retraining.

With the sale of Native American Air Ambulance (which, by the way, had already changed its name to *just* Native Air) to Omniflight, there were now a whole lot of new rules and regulations to contend with. There seemed to be no end of the line when trying to discuss problems either. With a corporation, there always seemed to be another entity to "consult." When you asked about something, your supervisor's answer was, "That'll have to be cleared with the president of the company." When you went to the president of the company, the answer was, "That'll have to be cleared with the CEO." If you went to the CEO, the answer was, "I'll have to put that to the investors." Or, "Put it to the board." Or they could always put it off to another department. "I'll have to check with HR,"

"I'll have to go through Financing," "I'll have to take that up with Operations." Always something. The buck just never seemed to stop. It was a convenient way to stall if not end the discussion. In my frustration, when a directive came down I always wanted to tell them, "I'll have to confirm that with the other crew members to see if that's appropriate." Yeah, but that's not the way it works, unfortunately.

One of the new directives was, you had to wear a long-sleeved black Nomex flightsuit and you could not roll the sleeves up because that exposed your arms in the case of a fire. You had to wear a full flight helmet. You had to be in the flightsuit from 7 AM to 7 PM, at all times, to decrease your response times. The notion that you'd be faster if you were already in your flightsuit. I timed myself one time and found it took me thirty seconds to get into my flightsuit and boots. Plus, we now had to wear helmets at all times while on missions. I once asked my Chief Flight Nurse at that time, "As a professional and knowledgeable RN, let me ask you something. Would you advise a person to wear full long-sleeved black suit and cover their primary biological radiator system, your head, with a hat and go out into the desert at 108 degrees? Would you consider that advisable? As a professional healthcare provider giving advice to a person in general." He just looked at me, trying to get my point. "Because that's what you're telling me. And not only do I have to go out into the desert with all that stuff, in that kind of heat, I have to work, lift, function, and think clearly."

The answer I got was, "Well, that's the way it is. It's to protect you in the event of a crash. If you don't like it, you know where the door is."

Well, I'm glad someone put some thought into this. Then

I realized I was just being bitchy. Resistant to change. But that wasn't the only thing that changed immediately after the purchase. Different paperwork, different procedures, different protocols, different mandates, and different rules. While it might have been best, certainly best for the corporation, it sure took a lot of the fun out of the job.

Chapter 25
POOR OL' COW

It was getting late one night, coming up on the time when we would normally retire to our respective bedrooms. We were sitting in the living area, Don, Bob, and myself, listening to Bob give us his first-hand experience of the first time he took a Viagra with his wife. The man just had a way to tell a story in that backwoods good-ol'-boy, down-home manner that kept you captivated.

"The dang thing kicked in and I almost lost my balance. I thought I was going to fall forward," he explained. "Heck, I was done and it still wanted to go. My wife started gettin' a little perturbed at me. I figured, hell, while I have this thing, might as well use it. She was all okay with it to start, but after a few hours, she was getting a bit tired of it. Well, I figured I'd give her a little break, so I decided to go take a leak and get something to drink. Thought I'd get her something to drink, too. That might give her a little time to get back in the mood, you know. But heck, I was having a hard time getting down the hall with the dang thing banging along the sides of the walls like a stick on a picket fence. *Tappity, tap, tap,* all the way down the hall. And the dang thing wouldn't even relax for me to go.

Dang chilliwhopper started shooting straight up in the air, almost hittin' the ceiling. Well, I tell ya, I'm shuffling around trying to get an aim, you know, a position where it's landing in the commode. I don't know what all I hit before gettin' it right. I know some went in the sink. Then, it was *tappity, tap, tap* all the way into the kitchen. I grabbed the bottle from the fridge and tried shutting the door. I'd swing the door in and it would stop and swing back open. Took me a second to figure out what was wrong. I couldn't get that close to the counter either, but at least I had somewhere to put the bottle cap while I poured us a couple of cokes."

Bob was animated and completely straight-faced telling us this. Not even a grin, he was serious. Standing up, pushing his hips forward, shuffling, mimicking everything. Meanwhile, Don and I were on the floor, tears were pouring from my eyes and I was gasping for air. But he just kept going on, completely oblivious to our distress.

"Well," he continued. "It's *tappity, tap, tap* back to the bedroom, trying not to let the dang thing slap into the glasses I'm carrying. Stiff as it was, that frog sticker would have cracked the glass ..."

"Native 5 scramble, Native 5 scramble for an MCA on New River Road," the Nextel interrupted. An MCA is a motor-cycle-accident. Nice that they made that distinction from an MVA. Anyway, same situation as an MVA. Who knows how bad it will be?

"Whelp," Bob threw up his hands and walked into his room to get his flightsuit on.

Meanwhile, I was trying to recover, wiping my eyes. I made my way into my room. Don, already in his flightsuit, quickly checked the map, grabbed what he needed and headed out.

POOR OL' COW

Bob and I were right behind him.

New River Road at this time of night was completely deserted. Truth be told, it was a deserted road most any time of the day. It was a rarely used road from New River, a small community north of Phoenix. Because it was rarely used, it was a great road to get out on and wrap your vehicle up to speed. Seldom patrolled, I have taken my Vette up there to let her loose on occasion. You just had to be aware that there were a couple of significant dips and two very sharp S curves. Not to mention, it crossed through a free range for cows that was protected only by sporadic wire fencing and cattle guards on either end.

They had us land on the road down from the patient. Once landed, we got out and started heading to the accident site. On the way up, I noticed a rather large cow about twenty feet off the pavement watching us go by. From the motorcycle pieces, skid marks and blood on the ground, I suspected that this was the point of impact. Everything indicated he struck the cow. I kept looking at the cow laying there, all by itself. It wasn't moving or making a sound, just laying there in the dark with its head up watching everything. Nobody around it. Everyone was down by the driver of the bike who I could hear hollering from here.

"I'm hurting man!" he is screaming. "Can't you give me something for the pain. I'm really hurting man." He was fidgeting around while the paramedics and firefighters were trying to get him secured on a spinal board. His cooperation in the procedure was minimal to none. It was obvious to any experienced medical person that the guy was in pain and, more than that, was intoxicated. It always kills me how some of the "tough" guys can be so wimpy in these situations. Always talking that tough shit, how big and bad they are, then when they get hurt they're screaming and begging for something for the pain. Yet how many times have I seen kids seven years old and women seventy years old just cringe and bare it when I asked them if they needed anything?

This guy had a broken arm that wasn't even penetrating the skin. Just a slightly deformed forearm that would feel better if he'd just let the medics splint and stabilize the darn thing. I was telling the guy, "Let us secure you to the longboard, get an IV put in and I'll gladly give you some pain medication and take you to the hospital. Work with us here. It's for your benefit." But trying to render care to an intoxicated "tough" guy is sometimes an exercise in futility.

We finally finished what needed to be done and got him secured to a spine board, his arm splinted and an IV put in. I hit him with a whopping dose of pain medication for his condition, which calmed him down, and we started carrying him off to the aircraft.

I was looking at the cow laying there, watching us as we go by. Quiet, alone, had to be in pain from the collision but not making a sound. The poor cow must be thinking, "Oh yeah, take care of the asshole who hit me. Don't worry about me. Someone will be along shortly to euthanize my ass because it would take too much to save me. I'll just wait here in pain until then. Yeah, don't worry about me, just make sure that drunk asshole gets taken care of. I'll just hang out here, thank you."

My compassion was for the poor "just minding my own business crossing the road" cow. My heart really went out to it. Meanwhile, even before we got to the helicopter, the guy was asking if he could get some more of "that shit." That shit being more pain medication. Having more help than we needed to load this guy, I stood back and let them do it. I paid attention that everything was in order and safe, but I couldn't help looking back at the cow one last time. Laying there calmly watching everything we did.

As we were lifting off from the scene, as explained, one of the critical times in flight, drunk guy attempts to sit up and ask for more pain medicine. I already gave him pretty much the maximum I could per our protocol. It was a significant amount. That, plus the amount of liquid painkiller he already administered to himself earlier, in leu of the extent of his relatively minor injury, I wasn't inclined to start pushing more into him right at the moment. I could give him another dose in about ten minutes. Bob, with a gentle hand, eased him back down, explaining the importance of laying still in a helicopter while lifting. Instructions that were readily excepted and complied with for almost fifteen seconds when he just forgot and did it again. Alcohol blocks short-term memory, a blessing for him and a curse for us.

Vital signs steady as a rock all the way in, with him trying to sit up every fifteen to thirty seconds, until finally, I decided that this guy looked like he might possibly get sick on us. So, I gave him slightly more pain medicine, completely within protocol, and a full dose of a fine anti-nausea drug called Phenergan. Just prophylactically mind you, because I certainly didn't want him getting sick. The "unfortunate" beauty of Phenergan is that it generally tends to make a person quite sedated, especially with alcohol in the system. Of course, if asked, that was certainly not my intention. It was just to keep him from getting sick. It worked like a charm. The rest of the ride in was relatively peaceful and uneventful.

We got done dropping off this patient and headed back

home to base. A pretty typical run at this time of night. No muss, no fuss, just picked up a drunk person who shouldn't have been driving, found out why they shouldn't have been driving, and took him to the hospital where they could get him patched up.

On the way back, my mind was preoccupied with the face of that poor cow burned into my memory. Those big blank eyes looking at us taking care of our own instead of the real, possibly critically injured living thing out there. The cow must have been thinking, "Fucking humans."

Chapter 26
DIDN'T READ THE BOOK

In the aeromedical business, you always have people coming and going from a base. Not as much at Native 5, though. We were kind of a coveted station. We were in the major metropolitan area, close to where most people lived. We had a reputation for being tight-knit and under the radar. What happened at Native 5 stayed at Native 5. But, on occasion, even we had a crew member move on and another one come in.

Bob decided to move on to the main office in Mesa to do the education and training for the company. In his place we got Mike R. We did have a lot of Mikes working for the company, so it was no surprise that we got another one.

Mike R. was a good replacement for Bob. Both were your down-home country types, commonly wearing cowboy hats when off-duty and baseball caps on-duty. Mike R. wore a baseball cap all the time. I think because he was thinning a little on top but still had a full, bushy moustache. Unlike Bob, however, Mike R. was a big fellow. Easily described as a great, big teddy bear. Easy going and gentle, Mike would give you the shirt off his back and his pants too, if you needed them. He was over six feet, weighing in at 240 pounds with an even bigger heart. His ideal Sunday afternoon was a big barbeque with beer for the whole family, and he had a big one. The man was no amateur when it came to slapping meat on the grill, that's for sure. He was a mentor and resident cheerleader for the Junior Marines, and every year volunteered for medical support at the annual Country Thunder outside concert event. He was another reason Native 5 was a coveted base. We were staffed with some of the best.

This particular night, I had Mike B. as my pilot and Mike R. as my medic. All I had to say was, "Hey, Mike," if I wanted to get someone's attention.

I was in my room watching TV and Mike R. was in the living area playing a video game on that TV. Mike B. had already gone to bed. At least, his door was shut and the lights in the office were out, when we heard the Nextel radio alert.

"Native 5 scramble, Native 5 scramble to Black Canyon City dog track for a GSW."

The dog track was an old abandoned area where they used to have a dog racing track years ago. Now it was just a weed-covered oval track, with old, ratty bleachers with a caved in roof and a large overgrown parking lot. It was in about the middle of the town, easy and quick to get to and the old parking lot was a great place to land the helicopter. It was often used as a rendezvous point. It was easier to have us land there and bring the GSW, or gunshot wound patient to us. Plus, we didn't have to worry about scene safety with firearms involved.

Gunshot wounds were rarely uninteresting. Unless it was a misfire, when someone tried to holster their weapon and the gun accidently goes off and the bullet goes down their leg, or something like that. Yes, that happens, I flew one of those. Most GSWs demanded a little thought process. If it wasn't immediately fatal, it could easily become critical within a short amount of time. It all depended on the area involved and the type of weapon used.

Tonight, we were in a different aircraft because Little Girl was down for maintenance. This aircraft was a B2 "A-Star." It was the one that looked like a dragonfly. The inside configuration was completely different than the Bell 206. The patient lays on the floor next to the pilot with their head essentially in the crotch of the medic, which made intubating impossible for the medic and extremely difficult for the nurse. Helicopters are very personal as far as close spaces. You do what you have to do to make things work.

We came over the landing zone and saw the one truck that would always meet us there. One of the town's elderly firefighters had an old-World War II-type military truck that he would bring out to sit in while waiting to land us.

When we landed, I went over to talk with him and see what information he had about the patient. He reported that this was a female in her thirties who had attempted suicide by shooting herself in the head. When I queried him, surprised that she was still alive, he informed me that not only was she alive, she was talking. Mike R. came up in time to hear that and we both gave each other a look of disbelief.

"They're about ten to fifteen minutes out," the firefighter told us.

Just about that time, his truck radio crackled, "Rescue 2, en route to the LZ."

He recanted, "Maybe, about five minutes out."

"Okay then," I said to Mike. "Let's get ready for this."

I was getting myself ready for a shit show. This ought to be interesting. A gunshot wound to the head. This was going to be crazy critical. Get ready.

About a minute before they arrived, we could see the flickering of red and white beacons lighting up over the trees in the warm night air, then the lights themselves, then the ambulance coming through the gate. We were standing out on the weed-covered pavement about the place we wanted them to stop from the helicopter. As soon as they did, we hopped in.

Sure enough, there was a female, about thirty years old, sitting on the gurney looking around very coherently. She had a head wrap dressing in place and a couple of IVs running. Other than that, and the monitor wires attached to her, she looked rather normal sitting there.

As usual, always start with a primary survey. The ABCs: airway, breathing, and circulation. With this patient, that was almost immediate. Her airway was intact, her breathing was good, and her circulation must be fine. She's sitting up, talking with everyone, completely oriented and with prefect recollection of the incident. She shot herself in the head, *twice*, the paramedic reported, with a .22-caliber pistol and never lost consciousness, either time. Twice, she shot herself.

With a head injury of this nature it is prudent to establish a definitive airway, in the event, which is very likely in this case, she stops breathing because of her wounds. That was on my mind. She's been shot twice in the head. Why isn't she already dead? Why is she still conscious? I had a patient before, shot in the head like this, but the bullet went in, hit the skull, deflected, went around the skull under the skin and came out. It never actually penetrated the skull into the brain. That was only one shot, however.

I asked her how she shot herself. Maybe not what you would think to be polite conversation. What any normal person would consider to be a question you don't ask someone. Actually, really personal and sort of prying. But I'm not in a cordial business, I need to know the answer. Using two fingers to simulate the barrel of a gun, she brought her hand up and pointed to her right temple. She made a motion like firing twice into her head. Pretty graphic. She left no room for interpretation.

"Never lost consciousness?" I reaffirmed.

She shook her head. "Nope," she answered. "Seems, I can't even do that right." She didn't sound sad or depressed but angry more than anything.

I asked her a few more questions, trying to gauge just how lucid she was. Every time I was quickly and deftly answered. I did a neurological check on her, had her squeeze my hands and let go on command. Had her push and pull my hands with her feet and checked sensations in upper and lower extremities. Everything was completely intact. Stick out your tongue, smile, blink, follow my fingers with your eyes. She responded appropriately. Pupils were equal and reactive and normal size. I peeked under the bandage at the right temple and saw two holes. I peeked under the bandage on the left side of the head and saw one rather large hole, about the size of a quarter. There was a moderate amount of bloody drainage on the dressing and the wounds were oozing but nothing too dramatic. All the time I was trying to determine if I should secure the woman's airway before we took off. To do that, I would have to "RSI" her; heavily sedate and paralyze her to keep her from reactively biting down. That, in itself, carries its own inherent risks. She is entirely too awake and alert to intubate her any other way, though. But how long is she going to stay awake and alert? It's not something I want to have to do in a hurry.

I looked at Mike R. with a querying look. "What do you think?"

He looked at me, then at her, then back at me. He cocked his head slightly and his burly shoulders shrugged. He knows the protocols too. Her GCS was fifteen not eight. GCS is a neuro status indicator. Our company protocol states, less than eight—intubate. I looked at the other two paramedics in the ambulance with us. They shrugged also. I was not really getting any help with this decision. I know it's about twelve minutes to the trauma center. I looked back at her.

"How do you feel right now?"

"I have a headache," she answered, unemotionally.

Yeah, well, that's a no brainer. Excuse the pun. Having made up my mind, I didn't want to waste any more time.

"Right," I said, as I stood up. "Let's get movin'."

Without any hesitation, everyone got up and started moving her to the helicopter. Because of the delay in patient arrival and time on the ground, pilot Mike had shut down the helicopter to save fuel. Also, it is always safer to load a patient cold, with the blades stopped. Not to mention, it's a lot easier to give and hear instructions. As gently as we could, we bounced her over the rough, worn-out, weedy and cracked pavement on the gurney. The old parking lot was such that as we moved along, the poor woman looked like she was on a vibrating bull ride, no matter how slow we went.

We loaded her in with her head elevated at 45-degrees, in a reclined sitting position. I really didn't want this lady lying flat. I didn't need blood pouring out of her newly acquired head vents. Or, worse yet, pooling somewhere inside her skull, pushing on her brain.

All secured and everyone cleared from the aircraft, our pilot confirmed we were ready.

"Hell yeah," I responded. "Crank the shit out of it." Just as I said this, I realized we were cold. No engine noise as of yet. Hopefully, just those of us with headsets hooked into the intercom could hear that. Our patient just had ear plugs in. Oops.

The whirring of the engine began along with a rather significant rocking of the aircraft as the rotor blades slowly swung around and came up to speed. Some A-Star helicopters had a tendency to rock pretty dramatically while the blades rotated around at the start. This one was more pronounced than others, at least, right then it seemed to be. But that could have been because I was a little more sensitive to it with this particular patient. I could imagine that the headache she complained of was probably throbbing. Though, when I asked her if she would like some pain medicine, she flatly refused. I would have liked to help the pain, but with her refusal I concurred. Not wanting to mask or confuse a declining responsiveness with head injury or narcotic effects. Nevertheless, I didn't want her roughly shaking back and forth by the aircraft either.

As we lifted up I noticed her vital signs on the monitor. They were staying rock solid in good ranges. She turned to look out the window, like she was just going for a ride. I started to relax a little. We would be at the trauma center in just a few minutes and then she would be their anxiety. I started charting.

I finished my chart in no time. Just had to add the name of who I gave report to, some times and get a signature, and I would be done. That was the game, get ready to go, be ready to go, stay ready to go.

We were still a few minutes out and I laid back to enjoy the rest of the ride in. It was uneventful in the cockpit with everyone quiet, just riding along. It was a nice night with bright stars to look at and this was kind of a cool call. Pretty unusual, anyway. I happened to glance at the monitor and noticed that her heart rate was starting to slow down, not completely unusual when a person starts to relax. But something about the way it was slowing down made me curious. Whenever I'm curious about my patient, the first thing I do is look at the patient themselves. She had her head turned away from me, looking out the window. I couldn't really see her face.

"How's she doing," I calmly asked medic Mike.

He looked down at her and exclaimed, "Oh shit!"

That's not what I wanted to hear. When looking at someone's face on an emergency scene, you can get three signs. The O sign, the Q sign and the dotted Q. The O sign is when someone is asleep with their mouth open and generally snoring. Not bad. The Q sign is when they're passed out with their tongue hanging out. That's generally an ominous sign. They're generally not doing well and you need to do something quick. The dotted Q is when their tongue is hanging out with a fly on it. That's a stable sign: they're dead. She was giving us the Q sign. No, that's not what I wanted at all. Crap, she was crashing. Just a minute away from the helipad she decided to give up the ghost. Shit!

Without a word being said, Mike grabbed the ambu bag, slipped an OPA airway in her mouth and started bagging, while I pulled out the laryngoscope, ripped open an intubation tube, and got ready to shove a tube down her throat. I could feel the aircraft start to flare back to slow down for landing. There was no way that medic Mike could get into a position to visualize an intubation where the patient's head was located between his legs. I unbuckled, slid over the seats and laid across Mike's lap.

Reaching over me, he pulled the OPA out and held her head in a position best suited for me to see what I need to.

To get the laryngoscope blade right where I needed it, I had to put my elbow on top of Mike's leg behind his knee. I could feel the pressure my elbow was digging into his leg. I knew it had to hurt but I couldn't help it. It's where it needed to be for me to control the scope to facilitate the intubation. To his credit, Mike never wavered his leg a millimeter, keeping it firm and steady for a platform for me to manipulate the scope. I was in an awkward position, lying sideways and tried to get my bearings in a completely unusual angle from a position that you never train for. I tried to move quickly, quicker than usual, because I knew in the next few seconds I was going to be jostled around when the skids touched down on the helipad. I saw my landmarks and slid the tube in just as the aircraft tapped the pad.

Instantly, Mike inflated the securing balloon and attached the ambu bag while I tried to retreat myself. We looked at the CO_2 detector to see it change colors to confirm placement. I listened, the best I could, to hear breath sounds on both sides of her chest and no gurgling, air bubble sounds in her stomach. I looked at the monitor for her heart rate; it was coming back up to her normal and the oxygen saturation was a solid 100%. While the aircraft shut down, Mike held the tube in place as he was bagging her at a steady, controlled rate. I ripped open a device known as a "tube tamer" to secure the tube in her mouth. Before the blades came to a complete stop, the tube was secured, her vital signs stabilized, and she was ready to move.

The hospital team was ready to come out with the stretcher and collect the patient to go in. The doors were still shut when I got my headset off.

"What the hell!" I blurted out. Mike, concentrating on bagging the patient appropriately, just shook his head. "I mean, jeez lady, you couldn't have waited just a couple more minutes?"

"Hey," Mike finally added, "when you got to go, you got to go."

We had given a report to the hospital while en route with our ETA and patient condition. GSW times two to the head, stable, vital signs good with patient awake and alert. That was not what they were seeing here.

"I thought you said she was awake and alert," the nurse said as we were pulling her out of the aircraft.

"She was!" Mike and I said in unison.

"What happened?"

Mike and I just looked at each other. Again, as if it had been rehearsed but hadn't. We replied, in unison, "She stopped."

The little nurse reached up to take over bagging the patient when Mike told her, "I got it." Not being rude, it's just that the patient was still in a reclined sitting position, on top of the gurney, and kind of a reach for the short nurse. On the other hand, she was right at Mike's comfort level. I told you he was a big guy, right? Plus, I don't think Mike wanted to trust anybody else with the secure placement of the tube. I was more than okay with that. He'd handle the tube and bagging and we'd handle everything else.

We rolled into the trauma room. The trauma doctor standing there said, "I thought she was awake and alert?"

Again, in unison, "She was!"

I finished my report with the usual, "Any questions?"

The doctor waiting for the trauma team to finish what they were doing in preparation, asked, "Just out of curiosity, do we have any idea why she did this?"

He knew I wouldn't have a reason for this. It was one of those questions that is often asked, even knowing the answer is unknowable. It wasn't going to make any difference in the care provided.

I shook my head, "No, sir."

He nodded, then, immediately, drew his attention to the team and started giving orders. "Let's get some blood for labs and get ready to go to CT." Which the trauma team was already doing.

My chart was done, now I'd have to rewrite the whole damn thing. "Well, that's a save," I said to the Mikes. We went into the EMS room.

"Yeah," medic Mike agreed, nodding slightly. "Just barely."

"Yeah," I said astonished. "What the hell?"

"Yeah," pilot Mike piped in. "What happened? Everything was going along quietly and then you guys just went nuts." At the time everything went down, pilot Mike was preoccupied with landing. A critical time in flight that absorbs the pilot's concentration. Even though everything is happening right next to him in the cockpit, he's so focused on what he's doing that he couldn't pay any attention to what we were doing.

"She crashed," medic Mike responded. "Just out of nowhere. She was doing good all the way up to that point." He looked at me with an apologetic expression. "I had just looked down at her before you said something and saw her blinking her eyes. She was awake and looking out the window. She was fine."

"Yeah, I don't doubt that," I nodded. "You know, in EMS everything is fine, until it's not."

"She was fine," he reiterated.

"No, I get that," trying to reassure him. "She just crashed. And when she did, she crashed hard. I think we were lucky to catch it as quick as we did."

"Well, what made you say something?"

"I just happened to notice the monitor, her heart rate starting to slow. I just happened to be looking at it at that moment."

"Well, I'm glad you did," he said, taking a drink.

Not wanting to waste any more time, I said, "Why don't we go down to CT and check out the scan?"

With that, we all headed down the hall to CT, which is located right before the elevators that go up to the helipad. The great thing about being the flight crew is the hospital staff is generally very accommodating to us. They tend to let us see things and tell us things that they don't ordinarily show or tell others.

I tapped on the control room door. It immediately opened a crack with a tech peering out. No questions asked, he lets us in. Standing there was the trauma doctor, two nurses, a couple of paramedic students, and the tech. Along with another tech operating the controls, the room was dark and sort of packed. I slipped over to the doctor and stood next to him, peering at the CT screen.

As the operator was going through the scan, I could see the bright specks in the brain that shouldn't be there. Again, being no radiologist, when something was obvious even I could tell.

Without looking over, I asked the doctor, "What do you see? Well, that's not already apparent just looking at it."

"It looks like just one of the projectiles entered the skull." He paused, stepped up to the screen and pointed at one of the bright pieces in the brain. "Can you enhance that?" he asked the operator.

He stepped back. "That looks like a fragment of skull," he said to no one, more just thinking out loud. "Anyway," he continued to tell me, "looks like one of the bullets went around the skull and came out. But the other one definitely penetrated and is still lodged in there, as you can see."

It was pretty easy to see the bullet. It looked like a bullet and was the shiniest spot on the screen. Because it was so dense, being made of lead, it stood out well around the other tissue. It was on the left side of the skull and there were several other speckles of dense colorations from the right side to the left. Fragments of skull bone tissue that had entered with the bullet. What the doctor was trying to determine definitively was that they were just bone fragments and not fragments of the second bullet.

"I can't believe she was talking after this," the doctor said.

"Oh, yes sir," Mike said quickly. "She was talking, oriented, moving everything just fine. Not airy a defect noticed. She was stable. Until just before we landed."

The doctor said, "That's amazing. Well, I suspect she's going to have some defects now."

We stood there a few moments longer. We'd seen enough. We thanked everyone and turned to head out. Just as we were going through the door, I heard the doctor say, "Good job guys. Strong work."

That made us feel better. I have to say, some of the coolest people you would ever want to know are trauma doctors. They may be confined to the emergency department most of their lives, but they see more than you could ever expect of life. Granted, most of what they see is the darker side of life. Trauma doctors are awesome.

On the way back to base, medic Mike and I, as usual, debriefed and discussed the call. Should we have intubated her before we left? It would have been appropriate and justifiable.

What could we have done different? Did we do what we should have done, when we should have done it? We discussed it. You have to play every case individually. Nothing is ever cut and dry.

We looked at this lady. We evaluated her. We did what we thought was best for her at the time, as it presented itself. We've read the textbook. The problem is, the patient has not. They don't always follow the textbook. Things happen suddenly in this business. Not just transport, but in every medical profession. Everything is okay, until it's not.

I have to give it to her. She did survive, and with a minimum of neurological deficits. Amazing. She should have died. Patients have just not read the textbook.

Chapter 27
MATT UHL

It was a nice day driving to work. I didn't have any crazy people driving around me on the way into base. The traffic lights seemed to be working in my favor, all green and the temperature was pleasant. Not a bad way to start the day.

When I walked into the base, the off-going crew and the on-coming crew were all sitting quietly in the front room. This was unusual but deceptively pleasant.

"Morning," I said. "What's going on?" as I walked into the sleeping room to drop off my bag and when I came back out, I was met with blank stares and silence.

Finally, someone said, "Matt Uhl was in an accident yesterday on the way up to Kingman to do a shift."

I seized up, like someone grabbed my gut and I froze in place. "Oh no," I responded, concerned. "Was he hurt?"

Again, silence. That, along with the watery, red eyes looking at me told me what I didn't want to know. It took a second to register, then I had to kneel down. I couldn't even walk to sit down somewhere. I couldn't stand. I couldn't think. Just silence.

"What happened?" I finally uttered.

"They called him to do an extra shift up in Kingman," I was told. "On the way up there on Highway 93, some car went to pass a semi and hit him head on. He died on the scene. From what I understand, they just pulled out right in front of him. He must have never had a chance."

Matt had taken a job working for Arizona Department of Public Safety, the state troopers, as a civilian pilot for their helicopters. Kingman, which is way up in the north-west part of the state, was not his normally assigned base. They had called him and asked if he could cover the shift, and knowing Matt, if you ask, he'll do it to help out.

I was in a state of disbelief. Not Matt. Not Mrs. Uhl's little boy. This was a person who you're lucky enough to meet once in a rare instance. A great husband, an amazing father, a terrific friend, a skilled pilot, and a fantastic person just to be around. Smart, easy-going, and humorous, you couldn't say enough good things about Matt. He was just one of those kinds of people everyone liked, for good reason. A rare individual. And now he was gone. Suddenly. Abruptly. Untimely.

Eventually, I made my way to a chair and sat there, sharing the stunned silence of my colleagues. We started reminiscing about stories of our time with him, being comforted by the mutual anguish we all felt. Before long, the off-going crew gathered their stuff and made their way out, hugging each other on the way to the door, not wanting to let a moment slip by where we didn't let each other know how we felt about them. Understanding the brevity of our time on earth.

Mike B. was the pilot today and Brian was my medic. We went about our morning duties and daily checks in complete silence. Of all days, this would be the one where we got a call very early on. An interfacility transfer from Maryvale Hospital to Maricopa burn unit. It was for a man that had sustained burns to his hands. Not very complicated for us. Not much to do, pretty much just load him up and take him to the burn unit. It wasn't a large area of skin burned, not life threatening, but burns to the hands are very complicated for the patient and need to be treated by burn specialists quickly.

In this profession, I try to keep my emotions muted. There's really no place for them. I used to be the type that would get pretty angry with drivers on the road. Living in a big city like Phoenix, you see some really rude behavior. Everybody's in a big ass hurry. Driving too fast for the traffic conditions, changing lanes sporadically just to get one or two cars ahead, and worst of all, driving entirely too close to the vehicle in front of them. There is nothing more dangerous than driving too closely. By far it is the most dangerous thing you can do while driving. I see it on the ground all the time, and I see it from the air too, just how many people do it. It's ridiculous. Then, one day, I realized that this is what gave me a job. I started looking at all of these rude drivers as my future clients. If they didn't become a client, they were going to create some for me. That changed my whole attitude. I didn't care how they drove now. You're not going to change anyone's driving habits no matter what you do. So, best to just sit back, enjoy the ride, and let them do what they're going to do. That's what pays for my house and food for my family. Just please, don't get all tangled up in front of me. Please, don't let the fact that you think you're the only person out here that has to get somewhere quickly, the only one that matters, get you to cause everyone else behind you to have to stop. Don't make me and everyone else have to suffer for your impatience. And please, for all that's holy, don't get me involved directly. Otherwise now, I'm cool with it.

As we were walking out to the helicopter, I was feeling a range of emotions. I tried to suppress them and concentrate on the call. I was feeling grief and I was feeling anger. This time, some impatient driver did get me involved. I had lost a brother and I was pissed.

We got in the aircraft, buckled up, and Mike asked if we were good to go.

Unsuccessful in holding my emotions, I barked out, "*Crank the shit out of it!*"

In that very instant, memories of Matt flooded into my thoughts. A flash of the first time he'd said that and how off-guard he'd caught me. Just by saying that phrase, it brought a soothing and tranquil feeling to me. It calmed me. Just what Matt would have wanted. It allowed me to regain my composure and get back to my normal self for a flight. It was just what I needed, I pulled out my chart and started filling it in. Yeah, I was back to mission at hand.

But then I noticed tears running down my cheek. Yup, I was crying.

The rest of the flight went along uneventfully and we returned to base. It was a solemn day. We got another ordinary flight later that night that had us returning at about midnight, and then we went to bed for the rest of the shift. In the morning, we passed along the news to the on-coming crew. They had already been made aware. In this business, information like that spreads quickly. It hit us all really hard.

From that point forward, every time I'd get in the aircraft and was asked about ready status, I would say, "Crank the shit out of it." It always reminded me of Matt. It was my way of following the edict of, "Do this in remembrance of me." That way I would never forget him.

As time went on, it became my mantra, "Crank the shit out of it." For just the passing of a moment, it brought me back to great people like Matt Uhl most of all, but also Rick Heape and the many more who have passed away in our profession. It kept me centered to the oh so many that I have flown with and worked with and have lost. It also made me appreciate those alive who I continue to share life with, depend on, rely on, work alongside of, and feel with. From the unseen dispatchers that are the first to hear the horrific screams of the traumatized, the law enforcement personnel that are first to unsightly scenes and strive to keep my crew safe, the EMTs, paramedics and firefighters that do the backbreaking and often heartbreaking and dangerous work to get access to those in trouble, to the flight crews that share my experience and help me daily, to the hospital nurses that take over when all is said and done. And, yes, even the doctors. That stoic, noble, highly-educated and extensively trained group of professionals at the top and end of the line. That, contrary to popular belief, I found out are *not* immune to the gut-wrenching emotions we all experience in this line of work. Yes, even they are vulnerable. They may be trained and conditioned not to show it, but in reality, they are susceptible. They're human. They are just part of the team, and they feel it. We are all human.

It isn't just a cute line anymore. It was his line, and I thank him for it and what it does to me every time I say it. I will always tell the pilot to "Crank the shit out of it." It's what cranks the shit out of me. It makes me reflect. It makes me think. It makes me my best. It makes me remember Matt.

Mrs. Uhl's little boy.

Chapter 28
GET PUMPING

Occasionally our flight crews were called to transport advanced technical equipment that the patient was on. These devices were only used on a few patients and it would be impractical to train everyone that transported patients in their use and function. Consequently, aeromedical was expected to be able to accommodate these devices with some amount of expertise. They were a smaller group of transport personnel that could be trained and practiced in the use of various kinds of equipment.

"Native 5 respond. Native 5 respond," the Nextel radio came alive. Along with other changes with the purchase of the company by Omniflight, we were no longer "Scrambled" on a call. That terminology was only used for the military. Now, we were notified to "Respond" to a call.

"Native 5 you're responding to Del Webb Hospital for a ventilated cardiac patient on a balloon pump, going to Boswell Hospital."

Bud, Brain, and I got up and gathered our equipment to respond to the call. We were one of only two bases that had an IABP device at the ready. They were expensive machines that were not used that frequently. The medical profession is very inventive with technology but not very creative when it came to naming things. A "Halo device" looks like a halo. A "Swan-Ganz catheter" was developed by Dr. Swan and Dr. Ganz. Some things were just called by what they were and what they did.

An Intra-Aortic Balloon Pump, or IABP, is a pretty cool machine that is a stop-gap for a heart in trouble until surgery can be performed. Commonly, when a patient is having a heart attack, they're taken to the cardiac catherization lab to have the blocked coronary artery opened and stop the heart attack. If for some reason the procedure cannot be performed or is ineffective, the cardiologist will sometimes place in an IABP to assist the heart and transport them to a hospital that can do open-heart surgery and just bypass the blocked artery. Its purpose is to help a failing heart. These patients are generally pretty sick. The hitch for us is that the device is about the size of a two-drawer filing cabinet and weighs ninety pounds. Which has to be lifted in and out of the helicopter after removing one of the back seats to make room. All of which delayed our lift off time.

With all of us working together, we got the back seat removed and the IABP placed in and secured reasonably quickly. It was something we did twice or more a month, so we were really quick at it. Once loaded, we cranked up and lifted off.

At Del Webb Hospital, we unloaded our stretcher onto their gurney, placed what equipment we were going to need on it and with Bud and Brian pushing the gurney, I followed them pulling the IABP on its own wheels. With security escorting us, we made our way into the cath lab and got a report.

This was a male, sixty-eight years old, arrived by ambulance about two hours before in a full-blown heart attack and was brought into the cath lab. He actually went into cardiac arrest on the way to the hospital and the paramedics were able to revive him before arriving. After inserting the cardiac catheter and trying to clear the blockage, they found that the angles through the vessels were too severe and there were too many coronary arteries blocked. He needed to have a coronary artery bypass graft performed at Boswell Hospital. On top of having the IABP device, he was also on a ventilator and several IV medication drips to assist his blood pressure, heart, and keep him sedated. This was going to be a busy patient.

He had five different IV medications running and all had to be delivered by an IV pumping device for accuracy. Each medication had to be programmed into the pump and specific tubing had to be used for our transport pumps. All of which took time. Once that was done, I had to program the ventilator and IABP machine. Once we placed him on our ventilator and our IABP device and moved him to our stretcher, we were ready to go.

I found it fascinating the way time could speed up to incredible rates when you're trying to set up and move a patient. It didn't help that this man had five different IV medications being pumped into him. He had a hose in just about every orifice and a few more in places the hospital created. He had a tube in his nose going to his stomach. An endotracheal tube for breathing in his mouth. A Foley catheter in his penis draining his urine. Two IV sites inserted, one in each arm. An IV placed in his neck. The sheath for the arterial line and the IABP catheter was inserted in his right femoral artery in his groin. This man had more lines going to him than my 1980s stereo system.

The man was a typical weight for us at 240 pounds. It wasn't that he was exceptionally heavy, but with all the critical lines running to him, he was cumbersome. All of these lines were crucial, so great care had to be used not to inadvertently pull one out. Once on our flight stretcher, we gave everything a few moments to make sure everything was working appropriately. Because the IABP is pumping and reading this patient's blood pressure with every beat, every time we moved him, or changed our altitude, the IABP had to be readjusted. Just another step that had to be taken with this patient throughout the transport.

With everything set and ready to go, we headed for the helicopter. From the time we entered the room to the time we left was about forty-two minutes. An exceptionally long time on scene for us, but in this case unavoidable. There was just a lot of stuff to do along with getting the necessary paperwork that had to accompany him wherever he went. We were moving pretty quickly but the clock definitely seemed to be moving faster.

When we got to the aircraft, we had to orchestrate lifting the IABP into the helicopter then the patient. The tubes and wires from the IABP to the patient were only about six feet long, which sounds like a lot, but it's not when you consider that this tether could not have any pressure put on it and could not be angled sharply or kinked in any way. Thankfully, the three of us had done this several times and were well versed in the procedure and pitfalls that could occur. Once we loaded him and the IABP machine in the helicopter, we hung the five IV bags on the two IV hooks we had, mounted the ventilator in its bracket and strapped down the IABP to be secure in flight. Then I jotted down another set of vital signs while Brian reconfirmed that everything was in the right spot and nothing had gotten pulled even slightly. Almost every line going in this patient was imperative and could not be displaced even a little bit. And because he was in such critical condition, his vital signs had to be recorded at least every five minutes. Once the patient was secured in the aircraft, now it was time for all of us to manipulate ourselves into our seats without disturbing any of these lines.

Once in flight, I had to readjust the IABP and record a new set of vital signs. I noticed our patient having a few abnormal heartbeats. Nothing I got too excited about, but enough to catch my attention. Our flight time was all of six minutes from lift off to landing. Six minutes!

When the device was operating, the IABP made a distinctive sound, with each heartbeat it inflated and deflated to, it made a *ta-pulmp, ta-pulmp, ta-pulmp,* sound. It was very noticeable when it was not drowned out by the helicopter. It should remain correspondingly rhythmic to the patient's own heartbeat. Occasionally, you'd hear it speed up or slow down and sometimes just stop. Any of these would catch your attention. As we were unloading the man, the sound of the IABP became arrhythmic. I heard the *ta-pulmp* go very rapidly and then stop for a second, then a couple more rapid *ta-pulmps,* then another pause, then a couple more quick *ta-pulmps*. I looked down at the EKG rhythm it was triggering to and noticed the patient was having a few more irregular heartbeats, more than I was comfortable with. By the time we had all the equipment out of the helicopter with the patient and ready to move, his heartbeats had settled down. The IABP became rhythmic again with a nice steady *ta-pulmp, ta-pulmp, ta-pulmp*. Funny how your patient's heartbeat can have an inadvertent effect over your own.

With our security escort, we rolled into the ICU with the patient looking like a carnival train of equipment. The patient, the IVs, the ventilator, followed by the IABP device, we looked like a rolling ICU coming down the hall and into the room, which indeed, we were. Even with all the ICU team and ourselves moving the patient and transferring all the equipment from ours to theirs, it still took about thirty-five minutes to get everything set up.

Now it was time to write the chart. This one was really going to be fun. Along with the normal chart with the extensive bodily assessment that would have to be done with this patient, with all the different tubes and lines and how they started and how they ended up when we left, there was a separate page for the ventilator and another separate page for the IABP. All the necessary vital signs along with all the interventions and procedures I did, not only to the patient but also to the equipment. All the checks for proper placement of all the tubes had to be documented for each time we moved him. The chart easily took more than forty minutes to complete, especially because I had absolutely no time during the flight to accomplish even a little.

All of this for a six-minute flight. But we got him here, all in one piece and none for the wear. I remember thinking, that's a save, as I walked away listening to the fading, *ta-pulmp, ta-pulmp, ta-pulmp.*

Every flight mission had its particular set of circumstances. Some you had to perform advanced procedures, some already had advanced procedures done and intricate devices that you had to care for, some you had to move really fast, which we strived to do each and every time anyway, but some you could be a little more relaxed with. There were patients that needed expert care and those that just needed rapid transportation. Every patient was different. This was one of the more advanced, critical and busy patients we would see. Not the worst I've had by any means, but right up there in the demanding category.

Chapter 29
EMS

For all the glory we get in flight for doing our job, and for some reason flight teams are glorified, I have to give it to the ground personnel, the firefighters, paramedics, EMTs, as well as the police. The police may not often be classified in the Emergency Medical Service but they are trained in first aid, they generally get there first and we depend on them immensely.

Now, our job is pretty cool, there's no denying that. But we're just a part of a big picture. A whole system that works together, from injury and illness to rehabilitation. We get to fly into the scene in a helicopter, jump out in our cool flightsuits, dash over and do our thing, and fly out. All very dramatic looking. Who's not fascinated watching a helicopter swoop down and snatch a patient and blast off?

But for every dramatic entrance that we made to a disaster scene, these ground crews saw hundreds more. They were the ones that got everything started, figured out the priorities, and rallied the troops. They're getting the patients sorted out, making the scene safe for others to come and assist, holding the curious at bay, clearing a spot for our glorious presentation, and cleaning up the aftermath, which, in itself, could be daunting.

Yeah, there were more than a few times when you would get exasperated with these people and their occasional arrogance. And I'm sure there were more than a few times when they'd get aggravated with our occasional swagger of superiority. But when all was said and done, it was the whole team that got the job finished. Hopefully, in the best interest of the victim of an unfortunate event.

Regardless of how anyone feels or acts in their personal life, I have yet to witness anyone's prejudice present itself when dealing with another person's tragedy. I'm sure it probably happens, it would be naïve to think otherwise. But I, personally, have never seen it, even when a patient was really being an asshole. Every medical person I've ever seen was just trying to help the person the best they could. Even for those people that probably put themselves in the position they found themselves in, medical people didn't care about that, they just wanted to fix them and get them better. It was a sense of pride thing.

On occasion, after a call, I'd have my team member say, "What the hell were they thinking on scene?" Or, "Why in the hell didn't they do this? Why'd they do that?" Almost all of the time it would be a valid point. They should have done something differently, or not have done something they did. Even I'd have those thoughts occasionally. But I'd just keep reminding them, and myself, "I guarantee, not one person was trying to harm anyone. I guarantee, everyone was just trying to do the very best they could and were doing everything they could to help. Plus, there are many different ways to do things. They may not be the way we would do them, they may not be what we think should be, they're just different. As long as it works and is not detrimental to the patient."

Every scene call was different. There was no book that

defined all the right steps to every scene call. This is very much a learn as you go profession. You're forever tested and critiqued. That's why you continuously train. Because, you constantly run into those scenarios that just hadn't been thought of yet. You have to work outside the box. The only way you can do that successfully is by working as a team with a lot of different ideas.

In most cases, everyone working a scene call had respect for all the others working with them. There were always exceptions to the rule, of course, but, for the most part, everyone worked as a team. I can only guess how many times I've relied on someone else at the scene for what they did only for me to get the credit for it later at the hospital. I did try, if I ever heard it, to set the record straight and give credit where credit was due. I knew clearly that the ones on the scene first could make my job easier and make me look like a star, and how others on a scene could absolutely sabotage me. They may not give you everything you really need to know in their report. Occasionally, some little tidbit would not get passed on.

"Oh yeah, the guy has a huge gash on his back" would get missed.

You wouldn't know because when you got there, the guy was already strapped down to the longboard. You don't want to waste time unstrapping him to check his back, as you really should. Plus, it's a little disrespectful, like you don't trust the paramedics on the scene. Then you walk in with the patient in the trauma room with everyone watching and the doctor asks, "What's this huge gash on their back?" And you're standing there wondering how that got there. Nobody ever told you about that!

I remember one time we got to the scene of a roll-over

MVA. A large SUV pulling a trailer had rolled over the side of a rather steep embankment. The sign on the side of the trailer read: "Bill's Gun Show" on top in a banner, and in smaller print in the middle "We buy and sell all types of firearms." The ground crew had already been there for over forty minutes extricating the guy, police had been there about ten minutes before that. They all had the guy out, strapped down on the longboard, IVs in place, the guy was essentially fine, just complaining about some neck and back pain with tingling in his feet. No obvious injuries but possibly some spinal problems that had to be ruled out. I got a full report, while my medic assessed him and got him hooked up on our monitors. We loaded him and flew him into the trauma center. My medic was already out of the room getting our stuff cleaned in the hallway while I was the only one left from the scene in the trauma room finishing giving report.

The trauma team was buzzing around the patient when suddenly one of the nurses exclaimed loudly over the clamor, "Oh, what's this!"

With a thumb and a forefinger, she pulled out a small, fully loaded 45-caliber handgun out of the patient's pocket and held it up high for everyone to see. Did the police that were on the scene first happen to check that? No. Did any of the firemen that extricated him check that? No. Did any of the paramedics that assessed him and strapped him down and put in IVs check for that? No. Did any of them bother to ask Bill from *Bill's Gun Show* if he was carrying? No. Are any of them standing here in this room where everyone stops what they're doing to look at me, the only one left from the scene? No.

What could I say? The only thing I could think of as I gazed up at the firearm was, "Well, that's interesting."

Would it be nice to know that the guy had a fully-loaded handgun on him? Yes. Would it have been a good idea to remove it and have someone secure it before putting him on an aircraft? Yes. Would it be nice to have that little tidbit of information when you're standing there in the middle of the trauma room sounding like the authority from the scene? Yes. Do you know what it's like to have egg on your face in front of all your professional colleagues? With everyone looking at you, Mr. Elite Flight Nurse? Well, you get the picture.

Thank you, everyone, I appreciate it. I love this job.

Chapter 30
THE WORLD OF TRANSPORT

Medical transport teams are a specialty onto themselves, whether it's in the air or on the ground. Aeromedical and flight crews are very much in the same realm as ground ambulance transport crews. We just use a helicopter or an airplane. I used to call it an ambulance with a rotor system. Aeromedical is a subsection of the larger medical transport system.

When coming to a scene call, a flight crew may have advanced equipment and procedure protocols that the ground ambulance crew does not have. That can make a difference. But flight crews also have limitations of room, weight, and where they can land. Airplanes have less restrictions on room and weight, but they cannot land on a scene or at the hospital, so they have to have a ground ambulance transport them to and from the airport.

When a person sustains a traumatic injury or has an acute medical issue, like a heart attack or a stroke, that's when the healthcare system starts. Generally, either a call to a dispatcher or a drive to the hospital. Whatever the case, that's when they step into the wheel of medical care. Technically, they should be the hub of the medical wheel that has many spokes working together to get them to rehabilitation and wellness. Transport is just one spoke in that wheel. Everything in this industry has its own specialty and most are not fully aware of what the other is responsible for.

EMS has its specialty, firefighters have their specialty, patient care technicians, nurses, and doctors all have their specialty. Labor and delivery, nursery, pediatrics, geriatrics, cardiac care units, intensive care units, emergency departments, they all have their own specialty too. Some have a very limited patient population, like labor and delivery. They only see pregnant people or something that has to do with that. Point being, you don't see male patients in that unit. You don't see adults in neonatal or pediatric units. Some have a limited scope of practice, like emergency. They see the whole of the patient population but they only deal with them for emergency problems, they diagnose them and then send them to the appropriate specialty care unit. Everybody has their place and does their thing. They all speak their own language and focus on their own domain. But they are all part of the team that gets a patient from illness or injury to wellness. No one is more important then any of the others. They all have their part to play.

Transport is its own specialty. They tend to see it all, trauma victims, OB patients with imminent delivery, pediatrics in respiratory distress, acute cardiac and stroke patients, and everything in between. Their specialty is in transporting people from one place to another. Either an emergency patient to the closest medical facility, or a critical patient to a specific facility that specializes in their particular problem. So, transport can be a mobile ICU, trauma unit, emergency room, a neonatal room, labor and delivery room, cardiac care unit or anything else. The difference is that it is mobile.

Often, I would come into a hospital to transport a patient and be told not to worry because the patient is stable at the time. "The patient is doing fine. Shouldn't have any problems getting them to the other hospital." Unfortunately, the nurses telling me this do not really consider the pitfalls and tribulations associated with transport. Why would they? It's not their specialty.

Of course, the patient is doing fine. Now. They're in a calm, climate-controlled, stable environment. They are resting and not being stimulated. Now, we come along and man-handle them onto a very uncomfortable stretcher, hook them up to all the necessary mobile monitoring devices, roll them around through the hospital, take them outside into 112-degree heat or drizzling rain, slide them into a transport vehicle, increase the noise level and vibrate them while submitting them to abnormal G-forces. Do you think their status might change? Most hospital personnel don't consider that. Again, why would they?

Because of the nature of transport, you have to have at least a general understanding of almost everything that can happen medically. In many cases, you have to have an advanced understanding of medical problems and situations. ICU personnel have to have a pretty good understanding of hemodynamics in a patient. How the blood moves around the body. Knowing about how well the heart is doing and the affects of the pressures going on inside the body at any given time. Transport personnel have to have that understanding too, but they also have to understand fluid dynamics. When accelerating and turning, how is the fluid inside the body going to affect the hemodynamics of the patient? Because of that, transport personnel are trained to notice and think about the affects of transporting a patient on top of the underlying condition to contend with. Like when you stop suddenly, all the fluid in your body is going to shift.

Our company set up and mandated clinical practices with our base hospital. Once a year, we had to go to certain units for eight hours to learn and maintain our knowledge of certain specialties. We had an OB, labor and delivery clinical day, a pediatric intensive care unit clinical day, and an OR clinical day. The purpose was for us to observe and practice specific skills unique to those highly specialized areas.

In OB, we learned and practiced examining patients in active labor and watched and learned how to deliver a baby. We had to read and understand fetal monitoring and drugs that would either promoted delivery or inhibited it. In the pediatric ICU, we watched and learned all the different drugs and equipment specific to the arena of small children. We saw and became a little more knowledgeable to different critical conditions specific to the pediatric population. In OR, we shadowed the anesthesiologist to enhance our ability to sedate and maintain a patient on a ventilator. We were also to practice our intubation skills by intubating live patients under the supervision of a seasoned professional that does it every day. It was a great learning experience.

The distressing part of all that is the hospital staff were not that overjoyed to have someone they didn't know come in and start doing their job. On more than one occasion in OB, I was essentially told to just stand in the corner, out of the way, and watch. Many times, in the pediatric ICU, the nurse I was following would talk to me only when not socializing with the other staff members and would give me the minimalist of information about the patients we were taking care of. When that would happen, it made for an incredibly long eight hours. Uncomfortable. I felt like an intruder and an outsider. Every specialty is very proud of their niche and protective of it from those not directly related to them. But, me being me, I would still insist they instruct me in something to further my knowledge base. Reluctantly, they would comply.

In our OR rotation, the anesthesiologists would always be hesitant to allow us to intubate their patients. Understandably, because they were responsible regardless of who did what if something happened. If the patient was not intubated appropriately, if a tooth got chipped in the process, or if the vocal cord was damaged during the procedure, the anesthesiologist was responsible. They really were not too thrilled with having someone they didn't know come in and intubate their patient without knowing their knowledge and skill level. They knew it was their responsibility to allow us to practice under their supervision but, I daresay, they weren't happy about it. It was a burden for them to mentor a stranger.

I had one anesthesiologist tell me, "I'll intubate the next patient and just let you watch." He looked at me contritely. "He's going to be a difficult intubation. I'm not sure you'd be comfortable doing it."

I quietly nodded respectfully. It was his show, I didn't want to impose.

"Yeah," I told him jokingly, not meaning to sound sarcastic, "this is completely different from what I'm used to. This patient is going to have had nothing to eat for over twelve hours, will be in a well-lit room, positioned up on a table, and I would be able to position his neck for the best possible view to intubate with. Completely out of my wheelhouse." I went quiet for a minute, then continued. "I'm used to having them after they just ate a hotdog and a bowl of chili, laying on the ground, gasping, in the dirt, in the heat or cold, in the dark, not able to move their neck at all and cars going behind me at sixty miles-per-hour. Yeah, your patient might be a little difficult for me. I'll just stand here and watch and learn."

I could tell he knew I was doing all I could not to smile. He contemplated me for a moment. Then he smiled. "Okay, I get your point. When he comes in, if you're comfortable with it, you will intubate. Let me know if you need any assistance or want me to take over."

The patient wasn't even a challenge. I'm not really sure why the anesthesiologist thought he would be a difficult airway, except for the fact that he was a big, obese patient. But, hell, that's most of our patients. I slipped in the tube easily and quickly, suitably impressing the anesthesiologist. The rest of the day he was telling and showing me all kinds of new tricks.

There is no unit anywhere in medicine that is more clannish than the OR, we were the outsiders and were treated as such, but the experience was enlightening. Getting a chance to have a seasoned professional, that intubates several times a day, observe and critique you practicing on a live patient was invaluable.

The challenge for transport personnel is how to utilize that ability to perform advanced procedures in the space about the size of a closet. How to perform delicate procedures while moving in a vehicle that shifts and bounces without prior notice and limits your ability to get into the optimum position to do what you need to do.

One of the things you learn to live with is the fact that you are directly involved in most of your patient's worst day of their life. In many cases, you are the human part of that worst day because they are so out of it. If you fly in close to the scene and take the patient out under the scrutinizing eye of any people who know them, you are the most memorable part of that worst day also. Every movement you make, every gesture you express, every grimace or smile that crosses your face is going to be noted by someone around. And, in many instances, you were going to be photographed or filmed, both by personal cameras and/or news media.

One day, my father-in-law had taken my son out golfing. We responded to a scene just outside that golf course and they were there, watching the whole thing. I wasn't aware of it at the time, I found out when I got home the next day.

Because of these associations you almost become the symbol of the outcome, good or bad. It's a feeling that you get that you can't explain to others. One of the things that always accompanies the worst day of a person's life is extreme emotions. Humans have a limitless range of emotions, all of which can be levied at you. When I am caring for a patient, I want to come across as professional but not so intense as to worry the patient or family. If possible, condition permitting, I try to be a little light-hearted in an attempt to lighten the mood and put the patient and family at ease. After all, they are being flown out, so the implication is that they already are very critical. But in the end, I've been hit with everything from, "I wasn't taking this very seriously" to "I seemed very serious and off-putting, didn't talk to us at all" to "I was so concentrated, how long has he been doing this?" It's hard to gage the reaction the family is going to walk away with. As a result, for the most part, I always came into the patient professionally, introducing myself and my partner, explaining why I'm there and telling them what I am going to do and what to expect. If they had any questions, concerns, or comments, I encouraged them to let me know because, after all, they were my only patient. I was there for them. By and large, the considerable majority were very gracious and appreciated the flight team coming in calm and easy-going. It did make them feel less panicked and sometimes took their mind off the situation, if only for a moment.

Over time, you just have to be able to read your patient, and the family if you are picking up at a hospital. I got to where I could tell when I needed to be strictly business and when it was appropriate to try to lighten the atmosphere. With kids, it's almost always better to be fun. Unless they're really sick and on a ventilator, then it's sternly focused business.

Why is it that patients who don't need anything want everything? Conversely, why are patients who need a lot are very appreciative of what little they get? When I get a little old lady, who has an obvious hip fracture, foot is almost pointed backward, and I ask her how much pain she is having, she answers, "Oh, it hurts some. But don't you worry yourself about it. I'm okay." She probably needs me to dump the whole narcotic box inside her. But then you get some guy who's got essentially the equivalent of a paper cut on his finger, screaming bloody murder, demanding the most you can give him for the pain. You just start to scratch your head.

That's when I started to realize that when someone is demanding that I do this and give them that, I know they're probably okay and going to do just fine. But when I get someone who is just lying there, not wanting to be a "bother," someone who is trying to *comfort me*, that's when my flags go up and I get busy. This is the person that needs my help most.

Someone flailing around screaming, "I'm dying! I'm dying! I can't breathe! I'm dying!"

Well, you're breathing well enough to swing your arms around and scream you're dying. Sounds like you can breathe, let me check you out.

But, when they're dusky-grey and say, "Oh, I'm okay."

No, you're not. YOU'RE DYING!

Now, that's not always the case, obviously. Sometimes when they're telling you they're dying, they really are. Get busy. And others, when they say they're okay, they really are okay. That's what makes this such a complex profession. You can't let your guard down because that nut job that's being a pain in the ass may actually be right. You don't want to be the person that walks back in to a dead body saying, "I guess I should have taken him more seriously." But after a while, you get more than just a "gut feeling" for these things. I can't put my finger on it, and I can't explain it. You just start to get a feeling, and your feelings matter. You need to listen to them.

In the world of transport, there can be an enormous amount of time doing nothing. When were not busy, that's a good thing. When were busy, that's a bad thing for someone. A team can spend a few minutes with a patient or an hour or more. But for the most part, there is a considerable amount of down time, that's why I say, when people ask what's the hardest thing I have to do, is trying to stay occupied between calls. Not that I'm complaining, there are far worse jobs. You had the ability to eat whenever you wanted, as long as you brought it with you, nap or sleep whenever, watch TV or a movie, play games, workout, or anything else you could do at the base. But, nevertheless, it could still get monotonous.

There is a true and definite need for medical helicopter transport. Used properly, it can make all the difference of life or death. Sometimes, it's not even that drastic. It can make the difference in salvaging a limb, or decreasing the severity of an injury or illness, or just increasing the odds for a better and quicker recovery. The reasons for utilizing a medical aircraft are huge. There are many qualifying conditions and circumstances, mostly distance and time.

All that being said, there are times and there are people that question the use of bringing in an aircraft to transport patients. Either from the scene of an accidental event or from one hospital to another.

I remember one day as I was standing at the nurse's station finishing my report when the doctor came up to me.

"You think you guys are overutilized?" he asked in a kindly manner. Obviously, referring to the patient we just brought in. Probably thinking that air transport was a little bit of over-kill for the patient's condition.

"No," I said vacantly.

"You don't?" he sounded bewildered. "Do you think you're underutilized?" I think he was seriously trying to get my take on the whole aeromedical transport reasoning.

"No," I answered. There I paused to let him contemplate while I finished a line. I stopped charting and looked at him. "I don't think we're overutilized or underutilized. I think we're mis-utilized. There are times when I bring in a patient like this, it seems air transport is a little much, at least I suspect so. But it's not my place to make that decision. I'm not a doctor, and realistically I can't make that determination. I also hear on our scanner about patients that are having a heart attack, or a stroke, and they get transported by ground ambulance. Those really are time-sensitive conditions and I wonder why we're not being called for them. It's a judgement call that I don't make. I'm not sure of the reasons. All I know is when we get called, we respond. When we don't get called, we don't. It's not my place to criticize anyone's reason one way or the other. There's times when we get called by a doctor at a hospital to transfer a patient to another hospital. When we get there the patient doesn't seem to be critical enough to warrant a helicopter. At the same time, I'm picking up that patient, I may see another one getting packaged by a ground ambulance that I think looks much more critical. But, I don't know all the particulars. Again, you call, we haul. No questioned asked. We just do our job."

The doctor just looked at me for a minute. I think he recognized the quandary we were in. He nodded. "I think I see your point." Doing what all good doctors do, he asked, "What do you think the solution is?"

"Education," I answered without hesitation. "It's really up to *all* the medical directors to establish guidelines for using different types of transport, and why. Then it's up to whoever picks up that phone to follow those guidelines."

The doctor nodded in agreement.

"But, then again," I added. "Every guideline is going to have room for interpretation. It's still going to come down to the one making the call."

I was thankful he approached me. It was a sentiment that I had encountered before by many others but was never consulted. He's not the first one that has ever questioned aeromedical transport. So, I appreciated the conversation. Was anything accomplished here? Probably not.

I have to say here; the world of EMS and transport care is not what it is made out to be in popular TV shows. On TV, every call is a life and death situation and there are many during a shift. The truth is that is pretty rare. Because of our training and experience most calls are really rather routine and there are not that many during a shift for most units. Most are run-of-the-mill calls that we see constantly in our job. Maybe one in thirty is a true life and death emergency that stands out in our mind as a traumatic event. There are some situations that we run into that the vision is impossible to erase from our memory. That being said, that equates to enough dramatic events that it can warp the mind of some in this field. That is why there are many with true PTSD and so many of us have an off-kilter, morbid sense of humor. It's what keeps us sane. The old folks in this business that are a little odd are actually the healthy ones. Far too many have been known to take their own life as a result of what they have seen. But, again, thankfully it is not an everyday occurrence.

The world of transport is its own specialty in and of itself. It has its own language, its own problems and its own solutions. Few medical people outside that specialty understand the full complexity of that little world. But it's okay, we know what we do and we appreciate the others in the field … and that seems to be enough.

Chapter 31
GOING DOWN

In our helicopters, on top of all the gauges that let the pilot know the status of fuel, altitude, attitude and engine perimeters and so on, there are also different navigational devices that assist them in spatial orientation and location. A map for aircrafts. Some of the high-tech navigational equipment found on aircrafts was not particularly user-friendly for the pilots. You had to push a button a couple of times to get it to the screen you needed, then you twisted a knob to scroll through letters to dial in certain waypoints, once you have the one you want in that place, you pushed the knob to move to the next space then scrolled again to get the three letters you needed in place, then push the button to input that information. Heaven forbid if you unintentionally hit the wrong button or double punch the right one in a vibrating aircraft. It will erase what you just did, reset, and you have to do it all again. On top of that, you still had the radios to contend with as well as maintaining the flight path of the aircraft.

A helicopter itself is a persnickety machine, forever trying to go its own way. It's been described to me by pilots that to fly one is like trying to juggle on top of a ball that's on a balance beam. You always have to stay ahead of it. One day, I was lucky enough that one of our pilots was ferrying a non-company helicopter to another airport for a friend of his. When we got off shift in the morning, he took my medic and me up in it to the other side of the airport, where they had a compass on the ground to check the accuracy of your instruments. Because it had dual controls set up in it, he allowed the medic and me to take turns at the controls for a bit to see if we could just hover and hold the helicopter in place. It gave me a whole new appreciation for what these pilots do on a daily basis. That thing kept trying to get away from me every second. Just trying to turn the nose in the opposite direction without changing our altitude was an exercise in concentration. It was easy to see how getting focused on setting the navigation panel, even in straight and level flight, could get the aircraft to wander off a little. These guys made it look easy and natural. And the places they'd have to set them down in the course of their job was a testament to their expertise. Fucking right on pilots.

Good ol' Bud. Yeah, he might have been one of our oldest pilots, if not the oldest, but I wouldn't hesitate to let my child fly with that guy anywhere. I remember one time flying along back to base with Bud at the controls. As he is preoccupied looking down at the navigation panel for quite a while, the aircraft was slowly gaining altitude. You could feel the forward momentum slowing down, as we were getting more and more with the nose pointing up. To alert the pilot, you might say something like, "Check your instruments." When you're high up and there's really no danger, sometimes a pilot can get distracted looking at something of interest. Not wanting to alarm him, I simply asked in passing, "Hey, Bud. Can you stall a helicopter like an airplane?" That was enough to get him to look up and correct the situation by easing the nose back down.

After he got back to straight and level flight, he answered my question as if it was just that. A question out of curiosity and not me telling him to check instruments. "No, not really. In a helicopter, it's known as settling with power." Totally cool and unfazed, he continued on for a minute, explaining the aerodynamics of settling with power, how it was like stalling an airplane but different. Then he went back to checking out the navigation panel. Unable to see us behind him, the medic and I were just smiling at each other.

Bud, Brian, and I were flying back to base from Thunderbird Hospital. Content after dropping off a patient with everything done and going back to quarters where we could eat. The call kicked out just before dinner and had taken about two and a half hours to get the patient from Wickenburg and transfer them to Thunderbird Hospital. It was late in November and already cool and dark outside. I had the side window open and was enjoying the breeze coming in. I loved flying along in the spring and fall with the window open and the fresh air rushing by. Periodically, I'd put my hand out to feel the pressure of 125 miles-per-hour wind pushing through my fingers. It was awesome.

We were in a direct path to Deer Valley Airport and could see our parking place from where we were. We were only about three miles from landing when Bud announced over the intercom, "Tighten your straps, we're going down here." His voice was solid and smooth, not alarming at all, which made it even harder to believe what he just said. Brian and I looked at each other enquiringly. "Make sure everything is secured," he followed up.

It wasn't until the helicopter started an easy bank around and decreasing altitude that we knew he wasn't kidding. Here?!

We're landing here? There's nothing below us but a parking lot. We were over a small shopping center with a Target store and an AMC movie theater on the end. The shopping center was on the southwest corner of the intersection of Loop 101 and Interstate 17. Two exceedingly busy roadways at this time of day. On the end with the movie theater, the parking lot was jammed full of cars with traffic moving in and through the area. Bud made his way to the opposite end, where the back part of the parking lot was vacated. No real traffic and large areas to land a helicopter in an emergency, except for all the decorative trees placed in the islands between sections. In Arizona, people love trees in parking lots to use as shading in the hot summer months. Right now, they were not a welcome addition.

Bud was bringing Little Girl down in what felt like a gentle, controlled landing, just completely unexpected. Suddenly, a remarkably nice and relaxed flight back to base had become very real, with our adrenaline up and now totally alert. Brian and I had no idea what had happened and this was not the time to question it. Pulling our straps tight, we directed our attention out the windows to assist Bud in landing in a place no one on the ground was expecting. When you're driving through a parking lot, trying to find that perfect spot, you're not anticipating a helicopter dropping down ahead of you. We let Bud know about any cars driving around the area that might create an obstacle or hindrance. Thankfully, there were none close.

Even with everything going on in a sped-up fashion, Bud was cool enough to key the radio and announce, "Deer Valley Tower, Native 5 making an emergency landing, three miles southwest, in the AMC parking lot."

Our home base was just three miles northeast of us, we could actually see it. Deer Valley Hospital's helipad was less than a half mile southeast of us, actually just across the street, but it was an arduous pad to land on in good conditions with buildings encircling it. Unknown to Brian and me, something was dictating a landing right here, right now. So, down we came with a perfectly delicate touchdown. As soon as the skids touched the ground, Brian and I hopped out of the aircraft to guard anyone from inadvertently driving into the landing zone or hard-to-see tail-rotor. Of course, putting a helicopter in the parking lot like we were just going shopping drew a crowd of curious on-lookers. Admittingly, not an everyday occurrence.

Once all the moving parts came to a complete stop, we went back and grabbed the barrier tape that we carried and cordoned off an area around Little Girl using those same trees that were a burden a few seconds ago. Before long, the shopping mall security officers came swinging out in their golf cart to see what was going on. We enlisted their help to keep any passers-by from coming up wanting to help. Everything was well in hand, except for the reason we were here in the first place.

After going through all the necessary shut-down procedures, alerting dispatch, and calling everyone else who was on the need-to-know list, Bud came out of the helicopter. Intrigued, Brian and I went up to him to find out the reason for our impromptu landing.

He looked at us, unfazed, and said, "There's something wrong with the tail rotor."

We went back to look at the tail rotor. Flashlight in hand, Bud scanned both blades up and down. He looked at the oil level glass on the side and noted plenty of oil in the box. He looked deep inside the mechanism as far as he could and pushed and pulled on the blade through its transition angles. Nothing. Then, he moved the blade to bring the top one down and check it. We heard a faint little *thump* come from somewhere in the tail boom. Not having any tools with us and knowing that this was now the realm of the AP mechanic, Bud stopped and just looked at it curiously.

"It just didn't feel right," he told us. "All of the sudden, I felt something in the foot pedals that wasn't right. A vibration that shouldn't be there. I felt I couldn't chance it, so I set her down."

"Well, glad you did," I told him. "I trust your instincts."

"Me too," Brian confirmed. "I hope it's nothing, but I would have hated to find out it was 'something' over the interstate. My daughter's glad you did too."

"Well, we'll just have to hang out here and wait for the mechanic," Bud said, sounding apologetic.

"Are you kidding?" I said, smiling.

By this time, a couple police cars pulled up and turned on their code lights to help secure the area.

"How often do you get to go to the store in a helicopter?" I asked. "I'm going to walk into Target. Need anything?"

Bud just smiled. "No, I think I'm good here." He headed over to talk to the police officers. Hell, being Bud, he probably knew them personally. So, Brian and I casually took a stroll into Target and checked out a few things. What else were we going to do while we waited?

We came back out a few minutes before Coffey and the mechanic showed up. Coffey gave Bud a "well-done" grin as he approached. He looked around, nodding. "Nice spot," he commented.

Bud cocked his head. "Well," he replied, "it was here."

They talked pilot talk amongst themselves a few minutes while the mechanic got his tools out and started unlatching the tail shaft cover. Turns out, about three brackets that hold the tail-rotor shaft along the top of the tail boom had broken. If Bud had of continued on, the shaft would have come apart catastrophically before getting back to base. It was possible for us to become a very expensive lawn dart, but for Bud's experience and expertise, we didn't.

I resolved from that moment on I was not going to give Bud any more shit about his flying. He had most probably just saved our lives. Whatever he did was fine with me. And I held to that resolve … for almost a week.

Chapter 32
THE HEARTBREAK

Because this business is the way this business is, you have ups and downs. It may just be what you have to do from day to day in your duties for work, like days when you're really busy to days when you do nothing at all. Or it can be in emotions. But the ups and downs can get pretty extreme at times.

There were times when several calls in a row would come in that may be challenging, may be busy or involved, not critical, just complex with a multitude of procedures. I've been doing this a while and lucky to have had great learning experiences in my career. Consequently, when dealing with patient situations, even as different as each one was, most are similar, even the hairiest trauma scenes always started with basic scene safety and primary survey with the first ABCs. The most complex interfacility transfers always started with the basic report and assessment. No matter how hard or involved any situation seemed coming into it, you just took a deep breath and followed a simple routine. Many times, it had to be modified for a particular case, but there were normal algorithms that you followed just as you've been trained and practiced. Putting all that with my experiences and it generally came down to doing what you did and have done; in other words, routine. But getting hammered daily was really rare.

Often, I'd have long periods where I'd either do nothing throughout the shift, waiting for a call, or I'd respond to a call. So, it all began to seem mundane, everyday stuff. Infrequently, we'd get a call that really threw something new into the works and you'd have to go outside the box and really think. Put all your experiences and skills to use. Not very often did we have to initiate treatments; more customarily we'd continue treatments already started with some adjustments and transport the patient. Shifts of back-to-back calls requiring dramatic life-saving procedures was really more TV than reality.

A sample shift was as follows: I'd transfer a pediatric patient, eighteen months old, that came in with a bad case of asthma, wheezing and having difficulty breathing. The hospital had given a couple of breathing treatments prior to our arrival and the child was doing much better, but they still wanted him transferred to Phoenix Children's Hospital for further evaluation and care. Easy call. The second call that shift was for a man who lived a long way out from a hospital, in his early forties, who had fallen from a ladder and broken his arm. An open fracture with bone sticking out. No loss of consciousness and no abnormal cofactors. Again, easy call. Splint the arm, start an IV, and give pain medicine to keep him comfortable until we got to the emergency department. The reason for flight with him was the distance he was from the closest hospital. The next shift I had was a shutout. I didn't do anything that day but try to stay entertained. The shift I had prior, I responded to a fall from a horse where the patient fractured her hip. Relatively easy assessment, with a shortened, internally rotated foot. She was a fit, mid-thirties woman with no complicating past medical history. With the assistance of the ground crew, we bound and stabilized her pelvic region, started an IV, gave sufficient pain medication, and transported her to the trauma unit. All business as usual.

The little "be-lep" of the Nextel radio chimed in and I stood up to get ready, even before knowing it was an actual call. Mike came out of the office to let us know that we did have a call way up by Cottonwood, north of us. That was a good thirty-minutes away so we needed to get going.

It was for a "pediatric versus motor-vehicle." When they put it like that, it generally means a kid hit by a car. It may be something else, but that's the first thing you'd think of. I had a doctor tell me one time, "When you hear hoofbeats, you think of horses before zebras." Meaning, think simple before exotic. So, it was probably a kid hit by a car, but that still left a lot of different scenarios. Not many of them are very benign. Even given the fact that kids tend to bounce much better than adults, their size, weight, and anatomical proportions lend themselves poorly to motor-vehicles. That, and the fact that they're so small, they're not seen sometimes, resulting in little to no braking before impact. All not good situations.

When we came close to the location, Mike contacted the ground crew to help us zero in on the scene and give us landing instructions. They were bringing us over a mobile home park and directing us to a playground large enough to land a helicopter, right across the street from the incident. We were also instructed to "bring the RSI drugs."

When they're asking for RSI drugs, it's a reasonable clue that they have an alert patient who needed to have a breathing tube inserted. Not a good sign. Especially with a pediatric patient. I looked over to Brian who was unstrapping the trauma bag, with the intubation equipment, in preparation for landing. Our intensity level just went up a few notches from already elevated.

On exiting the aircraft, we were hurriedly directed to the ambulance with its flashing lights. A man and woman, holding each other, were standing just outside the ambulance door, watching intently to what was going on inside. Staying professional, we climbed inside like we normally did.

The paramedic at the head of the stretcher was using an ambu-bag to give breaths to a boy lying there, with the assistance of the fire captain. The child's eyes were looking at me above the mask pressed on his face. He wasn't fighting the breaths, he was just looking at everything going on around him.

"We have a seven-year-old, male, run over by a big monster truck," the paramedic said. "His name is Tim. His information's on my chart, I'll give you a copy. He was riding a go-cart down the road and was not seen by the driver. The driver stopped after he felt a thump. Tim was alert on our arrival but was not breathing well." He nodded to the boy's chest where you could see clear tread marks going across.

He went on to tell me the boy had clear breath sounds on both sides of his chest but felt some crackling air bubbles just under the skin, indicating fractured rib bones. He was not breathing effectively when they got here, just gasping. His oxygen saturation was low when they first attached the monitor and his color was dusky.

Brian was attaching him to our monitors and running an automatic blood pressure. His heart rate was in the eighties and his blood pressure was over 150 systolic. A C-collar was already in place around his neck and two firefighters were finishing securing him to the backboard. The paramedic I was talking to was using both hands to fix the mask on the boy's face, while the fire captain was squeezing the ambu-bag.

"Other than the chest, was there any other injuries noted?" I asked as I grabbed a stethoscope. The heart rate had me concerned. I would anticipate a much higher heart rate, more reflective of a trauma and pain.

He reported that no other signs of injury were noted except for a large abrasion with a small laceration under his jaw. They were unable to insert an OPA in his mouth because he still had a gag reflex somewhat.

Now the paramedic looked at me, wanting me to confirm what he already anticipated needed to be done. Not wasting any time, I listened to his chest. His breathing sounded wet, with moist crackling heard with every bagged breath, not loud but equal and clearly heard all over on both sides. I looked in the boy's eyes that are staring at me over the mask. I popped the front of the C-collar open and quickly looked and listened to a couple other keys spots on the throat, which were harsh indicating air passing through a restricted passage, then I refasten it. Nothing was indicating a collapsed lung or air in the chest cavity.

"Are you having a hard time breathing on your own?" I asked the boy. I was asking for a couple of reasons. I already knew that he was having a hard time getting his breath. I wanted to see how he'd respond. Was it appropriate? Could he talk? When people attempt to talk they take a larger breath in preparation, could he do that? If so, how deep a breath could he take? One reply could answer a ton of questions.

Normally, when you ask someone a question with a C-collar on and they're alert, they try to nod or shake their head. Remarkably, he didn't do that. He just mouthed the word, "Yes," without making a sound. Again, more pieces to the puzzle. He was not moving his head as you would expect him to do and he was not vocalizing.

I asked him, "Are you in a lot of pain?" This time, again without any sound, he mouthed the word "Some." With him holding real still, not moving his arms or legs and not making sounds, it was a little hard to ascertain his level of pain. But with the despair in his stare and his poor oxygenation, it was not difficult to determine the next move.

"Yeah," I said to the crew, "we're going to need to RSI." That let everyone know with medical jargon, hopefully without alarming Tim or his parents that were standing at the door, that we were going to have to sedate him, paralyze him, and put in a definitive airway.

As Brian pulled out our intubation kit and got everything ready, I pulled out the drugs and started drawing them up. I allowed this time to address the frightened parents. "How much does he weigh?" I asked, including them in the care. They told me. "Well," I said in a soft, relaxed voice, maintaining a caring, professional tone, "Tim's having a hard time breathing. I need to put in a breathing tube to help him. I'm going to give him some medication to put him to sleep so he won't feel it and make him more comfortable. I'm going to shut the door because of the noise outside. Plus, this really isn't something you want to watch. You want to tell him you love him before I close the door?"

Seeing that there was no room to get in to touch him, they both yelled in from the door opening, "I love you! You're going to be okay. We love you very much. We'll be right with you. Love you!"

We shut the door of the ambulance. That decreased the noise level tremendously and had the added effect of taking what we were doing out of sight of the parents. Plus, it was a little easier to concentrate when you knew you didn't have the parents staring at you.

As I was already at the best position to insert the endotracheal tube and see the monitor clearly, with Brian sitting right next to the IVs, I handed him the medication syringes. With Tim being a pediatric patient, it was in our protocol to pre-medicate with Atropine, which keeps the heartrate from slowing down while I was poking around in his throat intubating. Children are more sensitive to that kind of vagal stimulation than adults. Plus, as I was looking at the monitor, I was aware that his heartrate was already slowing down at a consistent rate, but his oxygen saturation was maintaining at 94 percent, with occasional flashes of 97 percent. After giving the Atropine, Brian followed it with the pain medicine, the sedative and then the paralytic. Now I was hyper focused on everything going on, making sure the suction was on and ready, I looked at every piece of equipment I would need and where it was, while I waited for the paralytic to take effect.

Convinced that all the medications were on-board and working and Tim had gone to sleep, I had the captain give a couple extra squeezes on the bag then grabbed my laryngoscope and settled into the most optimum position I could get into so I could get the best visualization of Tim's throat. I slipped in the scope. I was not prepared to see what I saw when I looked into his mouth and throat. Children are notorious for being difficult intubations because of their size and the position of their anatomy. That was compounded this time with the fact that his head and neck could not be moved. It certainly could not be hyperextended to assist with visualization of the vocal cords. But I was prepared for all of that. What I was not prepared for was all the tissue in the mouth seemed to collapse in, making it impossible to ascertain any physical structures. I adjusted the scope down and then I brought it back some. Everything in his throat was moving, and not predictably. Things were moving in such a way to make it difficult to even predict where the trachea, or any other landmarks, where supposed to be. I was saying this out loud in the ambulance so the others could hear what I was seeing.

As I looked around confounded, Tim's oxygen saturation began to drop along with his heartrate, which didn't appreciably increase anyway after the Atropine injection. Dropping quicker than normal in this situation. I pulled out the scope, inserted an OPA now that he had no gag reflex, and started to bag his oxygen back up, which took more time than normally seen with patients, even pediatrics. Who are generally quicker to bounce back than adults. Once we got him back up to 96 percent oxygen, which was as high as he seemed to go, I attempted another look. This time being extra careful that I was not leaving out any vital procedure. A quick suction, going into the right side of the mouth, sweeping the tongue to the left out of the way, advancing cautiously, watching everything as I go, the same thing happened. Everything was strangely moving around unexpectantly. I was not able to even guess where I needed to be. I was not quiet about this. I was verbalizing everything as I saw it to the team. I knew I was not going to be able to intubate this boy and cut my losses before losing his saturation again. I pulled out, reinserted the OPA and start bagging again. This time he was even slower to maintain a good oxygen reading, and his heart started to slow again even with a constant saturation of 95 and 96 percent of oxygen and the Atropine on board. Atropine speeds up the heart.

By this time in my career, I have intubated hundreds of patients from my time as a paramedic, my experiences at Trinity Hospital, and my time in aeromedical transport. Not to mention the countless practice intubations on mannequins and cadavers. This was the first time I'd seen anything remotely close to this kind of presentation. I hadn't even heard about anything like this in all the years of discussing intubations with other colleagues. But all I knew right there was that this boy had to get a decent airway inserted quickly. I looked at Brian and asked if he wanted to give it a try.

Vehemently he shook his head, he said, "If you can't see anything, I'm not going to be able to. You've seen a lot more of these than I have." I looked around and everyone was shaking their heads.

On top of the pressure I would normally feel at a time like this, I was acutely aware that his parents were standing right outside the door. I could only imagine that every second we spent in here was minutes to them out there. I was sure every moment was sheer agony for them.

"Well then, hand me an LMA," I told him, holding out my hand. He had the appropriate size already laid out beside him and handed it to me. An LMA, or laryngeal-mask-airway, was a backup device that we used if we couldn't get a definitive endotracheal tube inserted. It was easier to insert because you essentially shove it down the throat and inflate a large mask-like thing on the end of it. In fact, the end of it looked just like an oxygen mask except it was up-side-down and cupped over the opening of the trachea. It's not preferred. The endotracheal tube goes into the trachea and, with a balloon, seals it off with the air tube going through the seal protecting the airway from aspiration. The LMA pushes up against the opening to the trachea attempting to seal it off and making the air force its way into the trachea, especially with someone like this boy, because with all the bagging, a good bit of air has gone into his stomach. Now, he's a good candidate for the pressure of that air in his stomach to push vomitus up the esophagus and the LMA isn't as good at preventing aspiration, or fluid going in the lungs, as an endotracheal tube. But it was a whole lot better than nothing in a pinch. It was better than what we could do with this child with the ambu-bag and a mask. It was the first time I'd ever had to use a backup airway device, and it was the only one we carried at the time. And I was in a pinch.

After having been trained and practiced many times inserting this device, I inserted it easily and it went in as advertised. Once seated well, I inflated the mask on the end to seal and started to bag air into the lungs. Every time I bagged, however, I heard farting sounds coming up from the throat, indicating it wasn't sealed off completely. I injected more air into the balloon mask with the same results. Another medic and I listened to breath sounds on both sides of the chest. Tim was getting air in both lungs but still had the unmistakable sound of a substantial leak at the mask down there. But it seemed to be working. Oxygen saturation was increasing, as was the heartrate, mildly.

"We need to get going," I said. Everybody took their part and we started to move the boy to the aircraft. I took a minute to talk to the parents, letting let them know we were going to the closest trauma unit in north Phoenix, and his condition. I didn't sugar coat what was going on. I didn't want to panic them, but I also didn't want to be misleading. He was in very serious shape, in dire shape, and I wanted them to be prepared. You have to be real, not alarming, but real. It's the only right thing to do. They had the right to know the truth. Their young son was critical in the extreme.

Unable to spend any time consoling them, I told them what I needed to and then got back with the team to expedite the loading. We got him secured, ushered away the ground team with our thanks, and prepared to get busy. Without wasting a second, we were launched.

Almost as soon as the skids came off the ground, I noticed the heartrate precipitously drop to nothing. Flatline. Zip. I reached for the drug box and pulled out an amp of Epinephrine while Brian got in position to start CPR. I injected the Epinephrine as Brian was doing compressions. Instantly realizing the situation, I notified Mike over the intercom that we needed to go to the closest hospital available, let dispatch know, and attempt to get the ground crew informed so they could tell the parents. I didn't want them to drive all the way down to Phoenix only to find out that we had to divert to another closer hospital.

The nearest hospital was the small Cottonwood Medical Center about four miles away. A couple of minutes flight time. It would have to do, this boy needed to be stabilized. Once we accomplished that, we could continue on to a more definitive trauma center. If the trauma center had been just a little closer, it would have been better to take the extra time to go there, but it wasn't. It was a good thirty minutes away. Too far to continue on in this condition when we might be able to at least get him somewhat stabilized. All the notifications were made and we were coming in hot.

Just as we sat down on the helipad, we noticed a return of

electrical activity on the EKG. He had a heartbeat again. Not great but beating.

The doctor and two emergency room personnel, along with a security guard, met us at the helipad and guided us into the emergency department. In less than a minute, we were in the emergency room, reassessing the boy and his condition. Almost immediately, he lost his heartbeat again. Another amp of Epinephrine was given and CPR restarted. We could all hear the bagging farts coming from his throat each time the respiratory tech squeezed the ambu-bag. The doctor announced that he needed to get a more secure airway put in. The LMA was leaking. I told him what I had seen in my attempts and was ready to assist. Along with his staff, he prepared to intubate the boy with an endotracheal tube. After less than a minute, his heartbeat began again and this time actually came up to about seventy-eight beats a minute and was producing a blood pressure.

Feeling a little defeated from my failed attempts to properly intubate this boy, I prepared to assist the doctor in his endeavor. He considered giving Tim a little more sedation but then dismissed the idea. It's one thing to be nice and compassionate, but in this case, not necessary. After the drugs kicked in and his heart was restarted with blood pressure and his oxygen saturations were back up, the doctor prepared to take out the LMA and insert the endotracheal tube. I held and stabilized his head and throat for the doctor as he pulled out the LMA and inserted his own laryngoscope to take a look.

"Jeez," he mumbled. "I see what you're talking about." He was quiet while he continued to look.

"His heartrate is dropping," one of the nurses said.

The doctor abandoned the procedure and stated, "Okay, let's bag him up a bit."

As long as Tim had a heartrate and oxygen saturation, he had a chance to survive. He didn't have to breathe on his own, we could do that for him.

The little respiratory tech put an OPA in and mask on, while Brian started to bag. The doctor looked at me with raised eyebrows, signaling alarm. Even though the boy's oxygen saturations were starting to rise, his heart rate really didn't respond positively.

Because Tim's heartrate remained low, the doctor ordered more Atropine to be given. That was done with the slightest of improvement in heartrate. Feeling he was getting about the best he was going to get, the doctor announced, "Let's try this again."

He attempted once more to look down his throat and intubate. Looking around and mumbling. "Why can't I see... What is going on... Maybe... No... Well, wait... What the..." Hearing the monitor beeps slowing down, he abandoned the attempt and pulled out. "Let's put the LMA back in," He said, looking at the respiratory tech. She handed him a new, prepared, readied LMA and he reinserted it, with the same leaky, farting noises after he inflated the mask to the maximum.

Tim's heart rate started to drop more. "How long since the last Epinephrine?" the doctor asked. He was told and another dose was ordered. He shook his head, looked at me, and shook it again. I grimaced and nodded, I knew what he was thinking, confounded, and I had nothing to offer.

This continued for about forty-five minutes. Tim would lose his heartrate, we'd give drugs and do CPR, get a heartrate back for a time, then repeat the process. Each time it was getting harder and harder to get the heartbeat back and after a while the blood pressure just wasn't responding. What heartbeats he had were not producing any blood pressure at all.

The only thing going through my mind the whole time was that when I first saw him, he was awake and looking around. I talked to him and he was able to respond. Granted, just barely, but he was responding to me and seemed perfectly aware of the situation and his surroundings. I was the one who put him to sleep. I was the one who gave him the drugs that knocked him out. I essentially euthanatized this young kid to get a breathing tube in him. I was the last one he saw, as he looked to me with trust to save him. I was the one.

After a prolonged period when his heart stopped responding to any efforts to revive him, the doctor announced that he was going to cease attempts at resuscitation. I was torn. Inside I was screaming, "Nooo!" I knew that we had lost the battle, but I was resistant to accept it. I couldn't let this be the outcome after the boy had trusted me to save him. My whole core was refusing to accept this outcome. He was too young. He was, in fact, the same age as my son. I couldn't let him go. Even though I knew the reality of the situation, I still couldn't admit it. What the hell did I do?

After he consulted with the team, the doctor stopped the process and pronounced the boy dead. I was devastated. Digging down and pulling out every stitch of professionalism in my being, I held my emotions. The doctor looked at me and asked, "Are you okay with this decision?" I reluctantly nodded.

I turned and grabbed my chart and headed out to write it. I told Brian I was going outside to write the chart and have a smoke to decompress. He understood and nodded.

I found the most secluded place available and lit one up, taking an enormous drag off the thing. With a great exhale, I went to take another and wasn't able to take much the second time. Unavoidably, I choked up. My emotions caught up with me and I could no longer hold them in. Now by myself, I let loose. *Bam!* Keeping a stoic expression, tears streamed down my face. All I could think of was, *I just killed this kid.* Such a young boy, and I couldn't save him with everything I knew. What had I done wrong? How did I let him down? What have I done? I was feeling an overwhelming sense of sorrow and betrayal to him.

I finished that cigarette in what seemed like seconds and lit another. I started to write my chart. When Brian found me, not saying a thing, he just sat down beside me quietly. I knew he was feeling the despair as well. We exchanged looks, but that was about all. That was about all that needed to be done.

"You need me to do anything?" he finally asked.

"No, I just need to write this chart. I don't know what to say. I don't know how I want to say it." How was I supposed to write that I just killed a kid? How was I going to write what we did and try to justify it with the outcome it produced?

"Just write what happened," he consoled. "This was a bad case. Just write what happened."

I looked at him. "What do you think?" I asked pleadingly. "Do you think we could have done anything different?"

He shook his head. "With what we had, I agreed with everything you did. What else could we have done? The little guy needed a tube. There was no other way to do it. If there was something else we should have done, I'll be damned if I know what it was."

My mind was racing a mile a minute. I was considering everything I'd ever learned. I was trying to think of any other scenario that would have changed the outcome. With all my years, I was at my wits end.

I went back to writing my chart as Brian sat there quietly. Occasionally, I'd ask him about a detail or something that needed to be added, just so this report was as complete and accurate as it could possibly be.

I was just about finished with the report, along with my third cigarette, when I noticed the doctor come out. I really didn't want him to see me sitting there smoking and writing. That didn't seem to bother him as he approached. I prepared myself to be professionally scolded and schooled. I was sure a doctor would have the compassion not to berate me in front of others but I was sure he'd feel the need to tell me where I went wrong. I was getting prepared.

Surprisingly, he sat down right next to me. He was quiet for a moment. "I bet you're feeling like shit right now, aren't you?" he said, genuinely sympathetic.

Unsuccessful in restraining a tear, I admitted, "Yeah. I do."

Sitting there, steadily gazing at me, he was not much older than me, if any. "I know there's not much I can tell you to make you feel better right now, but I need you to come with me for a minute." He patted my knee and got up. Compelled, I stood up and followed him, Brian right behind us.

"This was a tough call," he said softly, as we walked back into the hospital. I followed him into the emergency department. We turned a corner just before the room where the boy was laying, now with the parents standing there sobbing. Every whimper wrenched my heart even tighter. It was all I could do not to start crying myself. We went back into a darkened room with X-rays up on a viewing screen.

"I need you to see this," he said, stopping in front of a few images taken of a cervical spine. The X-rays of the boy's neck.

He pointed to an area just below the skull. "You see that?"

I'm looking at the X-rays. The second, third, and fourth vertebrae were displaced. Obviously displaced. I was able to make out the faint image of the LMA still in place just in front of them.

"There's the problem we had," he explained. "After they shot these films, I went back and looked inside his throat with the laryngoscope. Everything in his throat is swollen." He took a moment to look at me and then back at the films. "When he was struck by the truck," he continued, "it displaced his cervical spine. All the structures started swelling immediately from the insult. The spine, that everything attaches to, was loose. It was free floating. Nothing was fixed in place like it should be. When we went down to look, everything moved around freely and everything was swollen. He had massive neck trauma. That's why we couldn't see where to go. When you put in the LMA, it didn't work well. That's because the LMA depends on a firm structure behind it, like the spine, to hold it in place when you bag the patient. In this case, every time you bagged the kid, it pushed the spine back because it had no support."

He peered at me to see if I was comprehending was he was saying. I just stared at the films. I couldn't believe what I was looking at. I had seen a very similar scenario before. I remembered something like this a few years previously. There was nothing more I could do then either. I was dumbfounded.

"This boy didn't have a chance," he said. "This doesn't look like a survivable injury to me. This boy was going out, with this injury. If he were to have any chance of survival, he needed a tube. Without knowing what was going on in there, it was a hard tube to get. Well, even knowing what was in there, it still would've been impossible to get to. Unless, you were really lucky. And, if by some miracle you did get it, it would've still been a miracle for him to survive. His spinal cord is severed right there."

He looked back at the films and pointed. "No, I think you did this boy a favor by giving him something for the pain right away."

I know he was trying to make me feel better but it wasn't really working. He might have explained it, but he didn't make me feel better. Even though it might be a kind thing to do, euthanizing a dying patient, I was still not keen on the idea of me doing it. Especially a seven-year-old boy. It did help me come to terms with my decision and performance, that they were right, but I was still ripped apart inside.

To say that I euthanized my patient is harsh and a bit over the top, but that's how I felt, even if the doctor would disagree. It was not a good feeling, but more than typical with some people in this business because they're harder on themselves than anyone else could ever be. It's hard to be as detached as you should be. It can sometimes become far more personal than it should, but that's why people like me do this. We may grow a hard shell to maintain professionalism, but we tend to have rather soft underbellies that we don't allow the public to see very often. After all, we are human.

I asked the doctor his opinion about me talking to the family. He left the decision to me. I serenely walked into the room. I didn't want to impose my personal grief. They turned and I wanted to tell them how sorry I was for them but I couldn't. Every time I tried to speak, I choked. Tears fell out of my eyes, saying more than I could ever verbalize. Never knowing what emotional reaction you might get, I just stood there. Then Tim's mother walked up to me.

"Thank you," she whispered, with wet, red eyes.

I gasped and sobbed. "I'm so sorry," I managed to get out. "I tried."

She embraced me. "I know. I thank you."

I came in to comfort them, and here she is comforting me. Tim's father came over and put his hand on my shoulder and patted me, unable to talk either. We stood there quiet, sharing the pain between us. Eventually, I was able to compose myself enough to express my profound condolences. We hugged one last time and I excused myself. My emotions were crushed and raw. I felt overwhelmingly I had let them down, but they were completely understanding in the darkest hour of their lives. These are the moments that humble you and rightfully so. I made my way out to the helicopter. Mike and Brian were quietly talking. They watched me walk up.

"You okay?" Brian asked.

"Yeah," I lied, trying to shake it off. "You guys ready to go home?"

They nodded and the three of us climbed onboard. It was a long flight home with periods of silence and reflection. We were all spent from this call. This one was brutal on all of us.

When we got back to base, I called Susan and asked her to bring Sam up. He was my eight-year-old son. She kept asking me why. She didn't understand why I wanted her to get Sam and come all the way out to the base. And I couldn't explain it, but she brought him. When they got there, all I could do was hold onto Sam, with him wondering what in the world was going on. Susan went over and talked to Brian. I didn't say anything to Sam. I wanted to explain, but I couldn't think of how to put it. Plus, I didn't want to start choking up in front of him. It just wasn't something that he would understand, nor should he. That wasn't important. I just wanted to hold him.

Chapter 33
OUTCOMES AND RESULTS

We were flying a man who was seventy-two years old from Maryvale Hospital to the stroke center at St. Joseph's Hospital. While he was having breakfast with his wife, his left arm and leg became numb. He didn't pay it any attention to it at the time and decided to finish breakfast. The concern intensified when he said, "Weah, hat's oood," instead of, "Well, that's odd." His speech had become as slurred as a muddy creek. His wife then called for an ambulance.

When he got to the emergency department, they determined that he was having a stroke. Due to his symptoms and the fact that his blood pressure was 210/108 coming through the door. They started him on an anti-hypertensive IV drip and arraigned to have him flown to the stroke center.

A normal call for Brian and me, one of about 200 strokes I've done since I've been here. Really nothing to do but adjust his medication drip to keep his top blood pressure reading below 160. The doctor instructed us that he didn't want the pressure to go below 140 either. With a stroke, you don't want the blood pressure too high or too low. So, all I had to do was adjust a little now and then and watch him. Other than that, nothing to it.

We got him to St. Joseph's Hospital without any change in his neurological status and his blood pressure at 154/88. Pretty good for him. As was typical, we were met on the helipad by a security officer to escort us through the hospital. Usually, the security officer didn't know where we were supposed to go. I let him know that we were going to the ED when he surprised me by informing us that they wanted us to go straight to CT. So, they could do an immediate CAT scan of his head. That was unusual. Not that they wanted us to go straight to CT, but that the security officer knew that in advance. That was a plus.

It was about the middle of the day when we headed back to base. Being that the helipad at St. Joseph's is on the roof, Bud came with us to CT. As long as the helicopter was secure where it was sitting, the pilot would normally come with us into the hospital. In the summer, that was almost essential. You really don't want to be standing out in the heat that long. This being the middle of November, it wasn't so much the case because it was actually pretty decent out. It was a beautiful day with a mild temperature. It was the kind of day that I would comment, "That's why we live here."

We dropped down on to our spot at Deer Valley Airport and waited for Bud to let the helicopter stabilize and shut down. Like I said, it was a nice day and enjoyable to sit outside a little longer to relish it. Once shut down, the fuel truck that had come out to meet us came up into position to refuel the aircraft. Bud hung around while that was going on. Brian and I gathered our stuff and started to head inside.

Halfway across the tarmac, I noticed a young woman holding a child in her arms coming towards us. The man she was with hung back by the parked cars. It was not completely uncommon for someone to want to go see the helicopter, so this didn't catch me off-guard. Actually, it was nice when they came up to ask for permission as opposed to just going up without an escort to look inside. This was a nice day and she looked courteous and considerate of us.

"Hello," she said politely. "I don't want to bother you, but do you mind if I show my daughter the helicopter?" She was an attractive dark-skinned young woman, well-dressed and noticeably respectful. The child, maybe as much as two years old, sat comfortably in her left arm and stared at me with a cautious, quizzical look. When I brought my hand up to give her a little finger wave, she immediately turned around and grabbed onto Mom. That typical "He's looking at me, save me, Mommy!" reaction. Not screaming or crying, she just wasn't having anything to do with that.

"No, not at all," I replied to the pleasant woman. "Come on." Brian and I turned to accompany her up to the aircraft. We strolled up with her and the child between us.

"What's her name," I asked, trying to elicit a conversation.

"This is Ariel," she replied, looking down at her with obvious pride. "Bet you can guess how she got that name."

Well, that was a little unexpected. How would I know that? I let it pass without putting any thought into it. The little girl had turned around to watch where we were going, with an occasional glance at me with suspicion.

"It's okay, baby," she consoled her. "He's a good guy. He's your angel."

Again, a rather odd thing to say but nice. Not the oddest thing I've ever heard someone say about us. So, again, I paid it no mind.

They had just finished fueling when we came up and the fuel truck was pulling off. In the process of introducing her to

Bud, I realized I never introduced myself or Brian. Correcting that, I told her my name and Brian's.

"I was hoping to find out your names," she said as she moved closer to the aircraft. While Brian opened the patient door to let her look in, Ariel seemed to be one of those rare kids who was not intimidated by the aircraft but actually somewhat interested.

"See, baby," the woman said as she was checking out everything from roof to floor. "That's where Mommy was."

Now, that statement made me cock my head. Obviously, this lady has been airlifted before for some reason.

Curiously, I asked, "Have you been flown before in a medical helicopter?" Thinking probably when she was pregnant. High-risk OB patients are often flown to a hospital that specializes in that kind of thing. Not unusual.

She looked at me for a moment. "You don't remember me, do you?"

Now I was caught off-guard. I hate my memory. Should I remember her? In all honesty, most people don't realize when I see them, laid out ill or injured, they look totally different then when they're standing, healthy and normal. I racked my brain to try and figure out when I'd seen this lady before, assuming it was even me. Many times, when someone sees a flight crew member, we all tend to blend together. The flightsuit makes us all look alike.

"I'm Shanika," she said, like I should readily remember her name. When she said it, however, a slight memory started to stir. That name did sound familiar. It was definitely unique.

"You picked me up a couple of years ago from a car accident," she revealed. "I was pregnant at the time. I had a broken arm and a broken hip."

I looked at Brian and it started to come back to me. Oh shit! The "oh shit" girl. The memory slammed back now. This was the girl when "shit happened" with almost every part of the call. Pregnant, broken arm on one side, broken leg of the other, and everything we had to do was in a difficult place to get to. Brian's look changed from confusion to recollection right in front of me in that instant.

"Oh, yeah," I said as I beamed. "I remember! You look so different now. You know, not pregnant, not hurting, not all laid out on a backboard. You look great. How are you doing?"

She smiled. "Great now." She adjusted Ariel up in that left arm that was crooked and splinted the last time I saw it. "I wanted to thank you for the medicine you gave me. That got me through so much. I was so scared and you were so calm."

"We were just doing our job," I replied appreciatively. "You were pretty banged up."

"You were really banged up," Brian added. "We were worried about you."

"Well," she said and smiled. "Thanks to you guys, I did good. You're my heroes. My angels."

"Oh well, it wasn't just us," I said, trying not to let my chest puff out too far. "There were a lot of people involved. We were just part of the team."

"Yeah, I know," she confided. "They told me that I went straight into surgery. I was bleeding a lot into my leg and that had to be fixed in the operating room. They said my blood pressure started to drop as soon as I came in. It was a good thing I got there when I did. It could have had a bad outcome for my baby."

She propped up Ariel in her arms again, this time with pride, a little showing off. "It wasn't just me that you guys were taking care of. It was both of us. See what a beautiful girl you saved?"

I felt a lump in my throat. "So, is that where she got her pretty name, because she had already flown in the air?"

She nodded, "Yup. It came to me when I was in the hospital ready to deliver and I heard a helicopter. It hit me, that would be a great name. I asked Damon and he agreed." She looked over to the man standing by the cars and waved him over.

I looked over to Brian, we both had satisfied grins on our face.

"You want to get in?" Brian asked her.

"Sure, if that's okay," she replied enthusiastically.

The man she was with was walking over but had not quite reached the aircraft. I held out my arms to take the child so she could get in. Amazingly, Ariel, I guess having satisfied herself that I was no longer a threat, readily handed off into my arms. Now looking at me nose to nose, all I could say was, "Hey there, little one." Unable to respond, she just turned to watch as Mom climbed in the aircraft. Not concerned, not fidgety, just relaxed and confident in my embrace.

As her husband Damon arrived, we made introductions all around. He asked if I wanted him to take Ariel. I looked at her, with her being perfectly content sitting there watching Mom, and declined. "No, she's fine."

"See, honey?" Shanika told Damon. "This is where I was. Right here. Right here on this stretcher."

Damon looked at Brian and me. "I want to thank you guys for taking care of my wife."

"Our pleasure," Brian told him.

"I should say, my wife and my baby."

"She's a cute one," I told him, staring down at the beautiful little girl that was beginning to get a little heavy on my arm. But, for some reason, I didn't want to let her go, or this moment to pass.

We offered to let Damon inside and check things out also. Which he did after a little encouragement. We spent a good twenty minutes describing things, answering questions, and just talking. All the while, I'm holding Ariel in my arm. The two-year-old was getting as heavy as an eight-year-old, but as light as a dream come true.

"I can't believe the last time I saw you, you had a crooked arm and dislocated shoulder and broken femur. And pregnant! And now you're walking along perfectly fine, carrying that baby in the arm that use to be crooked and broken," I marveled.

"Don't forget," she added. "I had a broken hip too."

We talked a few minutes longer.

"Well," Shanika interjected. "We better let you go. We don't want to take up your time. I just wanted to come out and thank you for what you did for us." She took Ariel back into her arms.

"It was our pleasure, like Brian said, it's not very often we get to see the results of what we do. You just made our day. Thank you."

I'm not really the ooh-aah type of guy when it comes to kids. But, for some reason, just in twenty minutes, I had become attached to little Ariel and didn't really want to give her up. She was like a trophy, in an odd kind of way, that you didn't want to relinquish. And in handing her over, she seemed to have bonded with me also. How endearing.

We shook hands and then hugged. We bid each other the best and they walked off. Brian and I gathered our stuff back up, secured all the equipment, shut the doors, and headed up to quarters. Halfway across the tarmac to the hangar, I slowed and stopped. I turned around to look at the helicopter. Brian noticed it and stopped too, just to figure out what was up. I gazed at the helicopter sitting there emotionlessly ready and waiting to go on the next mission. Taking a moment to take in this rare contemplation of what we do. Yup, this was a pretty cool career. After years of doing this job, it sometimes became dreary and habitual. You became complacent to its wonder, neglectful of its coolness, it was just another job. It is something I do now but it won't last forever. I will eventually go on to other things. But man, it is a cool job. But … it is just a job. She was just one of the many that were forgotten in the blur of so many patients I have transported. That is reality.

With a slightly inflated chest, I was walking into the hangar with Brian talking about Shanika, Ariel, and the event that brought us all together. We were feeling pretty good about ourselves. This job could be tedious at times, like any job. Just because it was really cool didn't mean that it didn't get old. But right now, we were feeling rather invigorated. Yeah, maybe we really did make a difference sometimes. I was feeling pretty awesome, climbing the stairs to our quarters. When suddenly, Bud popped out of the door and started coming down the steps.

"We've got another call back at Maryvale," he said, passing by. "Cardiac, going to cath lab at Good Samaritan. Stable."

Well, that great feeling of accomplishment and boastfulness was short-lived. That overwhelming sensation of warmth and usefulness was rapidly passing as we took a deep breath. "Need anything from quarters?" I asked Brian.

"I could pee before we go," Brian said, obviously back to mission as usual.

"Yeah, me too," I agreed. So, we both scurried to the bathrooms. Him in the men's room, me in the women's room. No women around right now, so it was just another bathroom at that point. Then we hurried our asses back out to the aircraft, where Bud was finishing doing his pre-flight check. Brian and I buckled ourselves in and were ready to do it again.

Bud hopped in, buckled up, checked his list, and asked, "Good to go?"

I took a second, gathered it all in, then put my hand on his shoulder and said, "Crank the *shit* out of it!"

Finem Libri

MEMORIAE

Richard Heape
Matt Uhl
Shawn Perry
Mike Hanson
Lance Craig
Tina Alveraz
Janie Murdock
John Samson
Chad Frary
David Schneider

We raise our glass, adieu
For here is wishing you
Your skies, wherever
To be forever
Clear blue and twenty-two

AUTHOR'S BIO

Kurtis knew in the fourth grade that he wanted to be a cardiovascular surgeon. In that year he drew a life size skeleton of the human body and labelled each bone appropriately with their names. But life happens. He dropped out of school to joined the Army at 17 and became a combat medic in 1976. While there he obtained a paramedic certificate. After the Army, he worked as a medic and as an orderly in a hospital while he started to obtain his medical degree but, again, life happened and he ended up getting married and having a child. He obtained his nursing degree as an LVN then went on to get his RN. He worked ER, OR and primarily ICU before becoming a flight nurse in 1996. When Native American Air Ambulance started their first rotor-wing operation, he hired on with them in 1997. He stayed with that company until 2010. He continued his flight nursing with another helicopter program after that until 2016. After caring for his ailing mother, he hired on with another flight company after her passing. He continues to work in the Critical Care Transport field.

He currently resides in Sun City West, Arizona.
He can be found online at: www.kurtisbell.com
Email: anotherson@kurtisbell.com

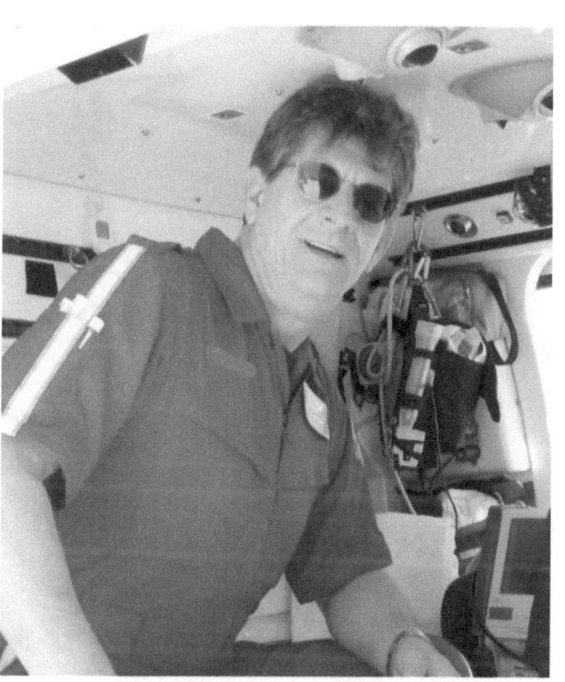

www.ingramcontent.com/pod-product-compliance
Lightning Source LLC
Chambersburg PA
CBHW020416010526
44118CB00010B/284